Linda Hume,
Nadia Khan and
Martin Reilly

Enabling Capable Environments Using Practice Leadership

A Unique Framework for Supporting People with Intellectual Disabilities and Their Carers

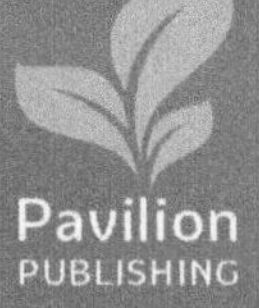

Enabling Capable Environments
Using Practice Leadership

© Pavilion Publishing & Media

The authors have asserted their rights in accordance with the Copyright, Designs and Patents Act (1988) to be identified as the authors of this work.

Published by:

Pavilion Publishing and Media Ltd
Blue Sky Offices, 25 Cecil Pashley Way
Shoreham by Sea, West Sussex
BN43 5FF

Tel: 01273 434 943
Email: info@pavpub.com
Web: www.pavpub.com

Published 2024

All rights reserved. No part of this publication may be reproduced, stored in a retrieval system, or transmitted in any form or by any means, electronic, mechanical, photocopying, recording or otherwise, without prior permission in writing of the publisher and the copyright owners.

A catalogue record for this book is available from the British Library.

ISBN: 978-1-803882-50-5

Pavilion Publishing and Media is a leading publisher of books, training materials and digital content in mental health, social care and allied fields. Pavilion and its imprints offer must-have knowledge and innovative learning solutions underpinned by sound research and professional values.

Authors: Linda Hume, Nadia Khan and Martin Reilly
Editor: Mike Benge
Cover design: Emma Dawe, Pavilion Publishing and Media Ltd
Page layout and typesetting: Phil Morash, Pavilion Publishing and Media Ltd
Printing: Independent Publishers Group (IPG)

Enabling Capable Environments © Pavilion Publishing and Media Ltd and its licensors 2024.

Contents

About the Authors 3

Introduction 5

Chapter 1:
Humanistic and person-centred approaches 9

Chapter 2:
Enabling capable environments 29

Chapter 3:
Applying capable environments: optimising individual and personalised supports 61

Chapter 4:
Sustaining capable environments – systems of support 85

Chapter 5:
The Periodic Service Review: moving from an audit process to empowering personalised practices 115

Chapter 6:
Practice leadership: Optimising a vision of practice 141

Chapter 7:
Person-Centred Active Support 167

Chapter 8:
Enabling Opportunities and Developing New Skills 193

Chapter 9:
Person-Centred approaches to understanding behaviours that challenge 217

Chapter 10:
Development of multi-element behaviour support plans 243

Enabling Capable Environments © Pavilion Publishing and Media Ltd and its licensors 2024.

Chapter 11:
The Role of Resolution Strategies 273

Chapter 12:
Evidence-based practice – what we should see 295

Resources 307

References 325

All of the resources are available online at
www.pavpub.com/enabling-capable-environments-resources,
from where they can be downloaded and printed.

 Enabling Capable Environments © Pavilion Publishing and Media Ltd and its licensors 2024.

About the Authors

Linda Hume

RNLD (Registered Nurse: Learning Disability), BSc (Hons), MSc, PgCert, FHEA & Doctoral Candidate University of Stirling.

Linda Hume is a registered learning disability nurse and is an independent academic and consultant. This also involves a post with the Challenging Behaviour Foundation as Coproduction and Engagement Lead, the Lead for Research, and Practice Leadership at the IABA Research and Education Foundation and a lecturer at several universities across the UK. Linda is also an Editorial Board Member for the *Journal of Intellectual Disability – Diagnosis and Treatment*.

Linda has worked in a range of leadership roles in health, social care and academia. Her teaching, research and consultancy focus on working with families, supporting organisations to understand and implement evidence-based person-centred approaches for people with a learning disability.

Nadia Khan

BCBA (Board Certified Behaviour Analyst), UK Behaviour Analyst (UKBA) (Cert), BSc (Hons), MSc, Doctoral Candidate University of Kent.

Nadia Khan is a Board-Certified Behaviour Analyst and is a Positive Behaviour Support (PBS) Manager at the Richmond Fellowship Scotland. Nadia has a background in adult social care, residential school settings, and individual support within family homes. Nadia is currently a PhD candidate at the Tizard Centre at the University of Kent, where she is researching staff psychological well-being within learning disability services. Nadia has experience working within one-to-one supports, as well as systems wide implementation of Positive Behaviour Support and has experience of conducting research within the learning disability field. She is a member of the UK Society for Behaviour Analysis PBS Significant Interest Group.

Martin Reilly

BTEC level 5 in Positive Behaviour Support from NHS Wales.

Martin Reilly is the Positive Behaviour Support Lead with the National Autistic Society in Scotland. Martin has worked with individuals with learning disability, autism and behaviours that challenge for the last 15 years. Over the last few years, Martin has focused on supporting the development of a national PBS team within the NAS and helping to ensure a consistent approach to PBS within the organisation. Martin has a keen interest in practice leadership, active support and capable environments as a means of improving quality of live and reducing restrictive practices for individuals supported within services.

Enabling Capable Environments © Pavilion Publishing and Media Ltd and its licensors 2024.

Introduction

Welcome to our book! We are delighted that you have chosen to read this book. *Enabling Capable Environments Using Practice Leadership: A unique framework for supporting people with intellectual disabilities and their carers* is written for anyone who has a role in supporting people with an intellectual disability to achieve their best quality of life, be that in the role of support staff, a manager, a commissioner, or an educator. It is also written for family members, so they might better understand what good person-centred approaches are and what they should look like in their endeavour to ensure their family has access to them. We appreciate this opportunity to share our collective experiences and knowledge of person-centred approaches and hope that this knowledge will inspire you, as the reader, to champion further the need for person-centred actions to improve the quality of support for people with an intellectual disability.

The purpose of this book

The purpose of this book is to serve as a core text which brings together contemporary thinking and practice in order to support an evidence-based approach for people with an intellectual disability and their families.

It is aimed primarily as a resource for health, education, and social care workers. However, it also serves as a reference guide for families and commissioners to benchmark personalised supports that indicate quality support is actioned in a person-centred way. This book sets out a unique framework (Figure I.1) that outlines the essential approaches that underpin capable environments and the essential requirements to ensure their successful implementation (practice leadership), focusing on embedding good quality support that leads to an enhanced quality of life.

The discussion and examples illustrate a contemporary approach to implementing person-centred approaches to help teams, commissioners and families develop a more collaborative, hands-on leadership approach and promote a culture of continuous improvement in the lives of people with intellectual disability.

We provide an overarching model of support to guide evidence-based practices.

Figure I.1: A unified approach to person-centred supports

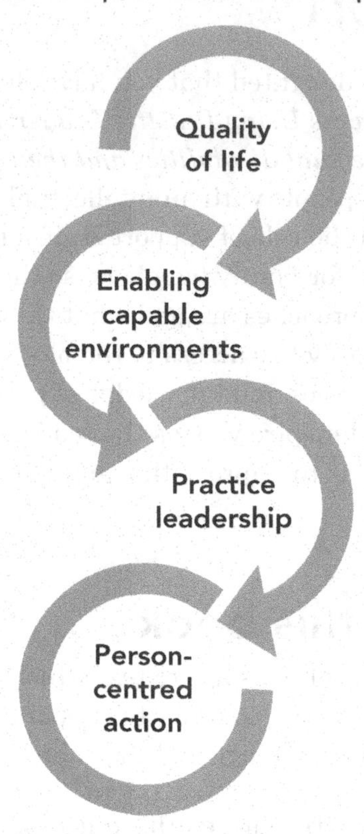

In this unified approach, an individual's quality of life becomes the driving force that leads to person-centred actions. Any person-centred supports are underpinned by enabling capable environments supported by practice leadership. This book will be the first resource to provide a more unified framework for how person-centred approaches are understood from the perspective of what a person needs and how such techniques should be implemented, supported and evaluated. It provides a clear and consistent message about what evidence-based practices should look like and how they should be appraised and evaluated in the context of quality-of-life outcomes.

This book aims to bridge the gap between organisational culture, leadership, and integrating evidence-based practices. It draws upon multiple person-centred approaches and provides tools and techniques that guide practitioners, teams and practice leaders to develop systems and structures to implement a unified framework of support that is influenced and informed by the quality of life of those who are supported.

Enabling Capable Environments © Pavilion Publishing and Media Ltd and its licensors 2024.

The structure of the book

This book is structured to accommodate several reading styles and interests. While the chapters are written in a logical order in which we recommend you read them, they are also composed so that you can access any chapter you are interested in. Each chapter will signpost you to other chapters that link to a specific topic as you go.

Every chapter follows a similar format, including an introduction, background and context, followed by conceptual framing, recommended approaches, implementation in practice, resources and discussion questions designed to spark additional reflection and insight from readers.

We are indebted to the people who have inspired our work, people with intellectual disability who have driven our practice and influenced our approaches, and their friends and families who consistently and supportively challenge our actions and remind us why we do what we do.

We hope this book is a supportive tool, enabling practical change at all levels of the organisations that endeavour to serve those with an intellectual disability.

Enabling Capable Environments © Pavilion Publishing and Media Ltd and its licensors 2024.

Chapter 1: Humanistic and person-centred approaches

'The role of the professional needs changing from being "expert" to being a partner in developing and delivering individualised supports.' (Buntinx, 2015)

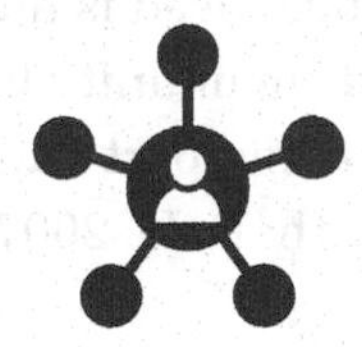

Chapter contents:

- Understanding the concept and history of a humanistic approach to support for people with intellectual disabilities.
- A discussion on the quality-of-life domains.
- Understanding the need for person-centred action in service planning and delivery.
- The principles of person-centred approaches.
- The rationale for a unified approach.

Learning outcomes

After reading this chapter and completing the suggested activities and reflection, the reader should be able to:

- Recognise how models of support are used in the design of services for people with intellectual disabilities.
- Identify the underpinning principles of individualised personalised support.
- Develop an understanding of how quality-of-life domains are translated into person-centred actions.
- Align their practice to a unified approach focused on person-centred support.

Introduction

Humanistic principles describe the attitudes and behaviours that demonstrate an interest in and respect for people's social and psychological well-being. People's actions should, therefore, be aligned with these beliefs and values, and our perspectives should be rooted in a strengths-based approach.

This shift to more humanistic and ecological approaches aims to move the focus of professional support from diagnosis and identifying what someone cannot do, to a broader focus on assessing and supporting strengths and providing opportunities and resources to enhance people's quality of life. This perspective shift was presented by Schalock *et al.* (2010) who proposed the need for a system that recognises that the support people need is not specialist and inaccessible but that these supports are generic, and community based. This need for more well-developed and responsive community support had already been identified in the UK by Mansell (Department of Health: DoH, 2007).

> *'Often, community-based services have not been sufficiently well-developed and well-organised to serve [people with learning disabilities]. Placements break down as people whose behaviour presents a challenge can no longer be supported.'* (DoH, 2007)

However, it seems that specialist support is still beyond the reach of people with intellectual disability at the point when they need it because of tiers and silos and pathways, which create barriers to access. In 2020, the Challenging Behaviour Foundation (CBF) surveyed family members, exploring their experiences navigating the systems supporting their family members. The report was titled *Broken* with the subheading: 'The system is broken, and no one takes any responsibility'. As part of this research, families identified the risk factors that they thought increased the likelihood of trauma for them. These included:

- Lack of services and support to meet my relative's individual needs (81%).
- Lack of early intervention services and support (77%).
- Lack of specialist support, i.e., trained staff/support workers with intellectual disability experience (76%).
- Finding a way through the education, health, and social care system (71%) (*Broken*, p10).

Enabling Capable Environments © Pavilion Publishing and Media Ltd and its licensors 2024.

One family member described their experience of trying to access support as follows:

'I feel that paid professionals only seem to be brought in when a crisis has already happened. This is usually too far down the line. We, as a family, highlighted our relative's declining situation 18 months before they got sent miles away in a knee-jerk reaction as it was two weeks before Christmas and was the only bed available' (CBF, 2020, p14).

Reports of dissatisfaction with services for people with an intellectual disability remain common. This dissatisfaction can range from poorly rated inspection reports from external bodies, where parts of the systems and processes of an organisation need to meet agreed criteria and require improvement. It can also reflect a system that not only does not 'care' but is systematic in the neglect and abuse of people with an intellectual disability, which can result in catastrophic consequences for individuals and their families; Winterbourne View (*Undercover Care: The Abuse Exposed, 2011), Whorlton Hall (*Undercover Hospital Abuse Scandal, 2019), and Muckamore Abbey (BBC News, 2020). While these may appear as exceptional examples of services that are not fit for purpose, they reflect a journey of systematic failings at multiple levels.

The lack of consideration for people's needs can also be reflected in the daily lives of people with an intellectual disability as they attempt to navigate a system which is meant to support them but instead responds not only with a lack of compassion and understanding but, due to factors such as diagnostic overshadowing, can put people at risk of harm (for example, changes to someone's presentation being misattributed to their intellectual disability and not an indicator that their basic needs should be reviewed for physical health conditions). People with an intellectual disability are overprescribed medications such as psychotropic medications. These factors and many others are found in the *Learning Disabilities Mortality Review* (LeDeR: 2021) Programme, and Mencap's *Death by Indifference Report* (2007). Despite the banner of person centred care, what people with an intellectual disability face is dehumanising care that is not holistic or responsive to their current needs.

Models of support and quality of life

There is no overarching model of support for learning/intellectual disability services, however, one of the key factors should be the concept of quality of life – that there should be a clear and consistent message that services and staff teams should put the individual's quality of life outcomes at the centre of everything they do (DoH, 2007).

There is a need for services to adopt a strengths-based focus and while perspectives of quality of life can be subjective, it is important to acknowledge that one single framework will not fully address the complexity of embedding these domains into practice. Humanistic approaches to support delivery require a more multi-dimensional approach which is outlined in the quality-of-life domains identified by Schalock *et al*. (2010).

Quality of life is a key premise of policy guidance within services for people with an intellectual disability. The concept of quality of life includes:

- Fostering the provision of individualised support.
- Furthering the development of evidence-based practices.
- Encouraging the evaluation of personal outcomes.
- Providing a quality framework for continuous quality improvement.

These points should be the driving factors behind how support for people with an intellectual disability is organised and delivered (Schalock & Alonso, 2015).

Research has demonstrated that quality-of-life outcomes and quality of support are key variables in services, particularly for people with more complex needs such as challenging behaviour (Bigby & Beadle-Brown, 2016). Schalock *et al*. (2002) summarised quality of life as having eight domains: emotional well-being, interpersonal relations, material well-being, personal development, physical well-being, self-determination, social inclusion, and rights.

Table 1.1: Quality-of-life domains (Schalock *et al.*, 2002)

Domain	Indicators
Emotional well-being	Contentment, lack of stress, level of challenging behaviour
Interpersonal relations	Interactions, relationships, supports
Material well-being	Financial status, employment and housing
Personal development	Education, opportunities for participating in activities and developing skills

 Enabling Capable Environments © Pavilion Publishing and Media Ltd and its licensors 2024.

Physical well-being	Health and healthcare, activities of daily living and leisure
Self-determination	Autonomy, personal control, goals and personal values and choices
Social inclusion	Community integration and participation in community roles and social supports
Rights	Human, respect, dignity, equality and legal

Emotional well-being

Emotional well-being is considered a state of being in which you have a sense of balance, positivity, and contentment in your life; the ability to pursue things and people that make you happy. There are several ways to think about emotional well-being, but it is important to recognise that it is more than just *being happy*. It needs to be considered in the context of the individual and it must be a driving outcome of any service support. We have drawn upon a model from Ryff (1989) to illustrate that emotional well-being is multifaced and dynamic.

Figure 1.1: Dimensions of emotional well-being

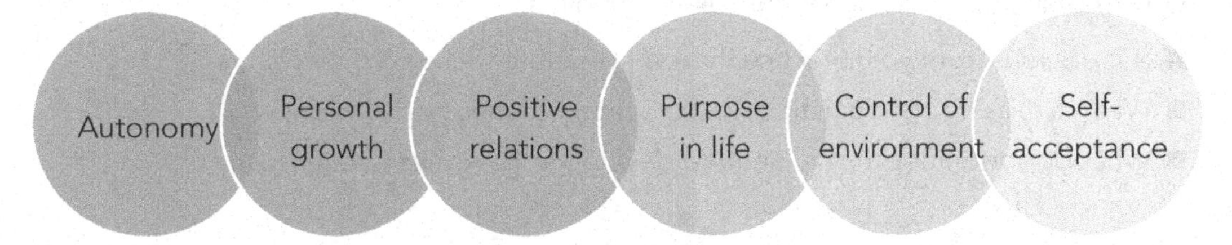

Let's look at each of these dimensions:

- **Autonomy:** The person is independent and acts independently of social pressures. An example of this might be: 'I have confidence in my opinions, even if they are contrary to the consensus'.
- **Personal growth:** The person continues to develop, accessing new experiences and self-development over time. An example of this might be: 'I think it is important to have new experiences that challenge how I think about myself and the world'.
- **Positive relations with others:** This reflects the person's engagement in meaningful relationships that include reciprocal empathy, intimacy and

affection. An example might be: 'I feel that people like me, and I have a circle of friends'.

- **Purpose in life:** The person has a strong goal orientation and conviction that life holds meaning. An example might be: 'I have a sense of direction and purpose in my life'.
- **Control of environment:** The person can effectively use opportunities and has influence over environmental factors and activities, including managing everyday affairs and creating situations to meet their personal needs. An example could be: 'In general, I feel I am in charge of the situation in which I live'.
- **Self-acceptance:** The person has a positive attitude about themselves. An example of this might be: 'I like most aspects of my life and am proud of who I am'.

Thinking space

Each dimension in this model is explained above. As a reflective exercise, consider how each of the dimensions of emotional well-being (Figure 1.1) are explicit in your day-to-day practice.

For each dimension consider the following points:

- Is it obvious from your practice that you promote these six dimensions?
- What is missing from practices in the context of these dimensions?
- What opportunities do you need to develop skills in these areas?

Interpersonal relations

Schalock & Verdugo (2015) define interpersonal relationships as having a close circle of friends, family involvement and natural support, i.e. people who are not paid to be with the person. However, research shows that people with an intellectual disability experience difficulties with developing relationships, with people with severe intellectual disabilities being more significantly disadvantaged. Research by Johnson *et al.* (2012) showed that, at times, paid staff provided limited opportunities for people with an intellectual disability for social interaction and that in adult service provision, contact with paid staff is infrequent and can be more task or instruction-driven rather than relationship-driven.

 Enabling Capable Environments © Pavilion Publishing and Media Ltd and its licensors 2024.

This does lead us to question if this domain of interpersonal relationships is made explicit in job descriptions. Are people provided with training to facilitate the development of relationships? If the answer is no to these questions, there is a risk that the development of relationships is left to chance and seen as a low priority.

We return to the study by Johnston *et al.* (2012) for two reasons. First, it is an essential contribution to the research that, importantly, captures the views of people with intellectual disabilities. Secondly, the article title, which includes the terms 'Having Fun and Hanging Out', certainly warrants further reading.

In this study, the authors present a theory (based on interviews with people with an intellectual disability). The overarching theme of this theory is sharing the moment, with sub-themes including, as per the title, *hanging out and having fun*; these signify the diversity of friendship and relationships that are often overlooked as key indicators of quality of life.

Figure 1.1: Relationship themes

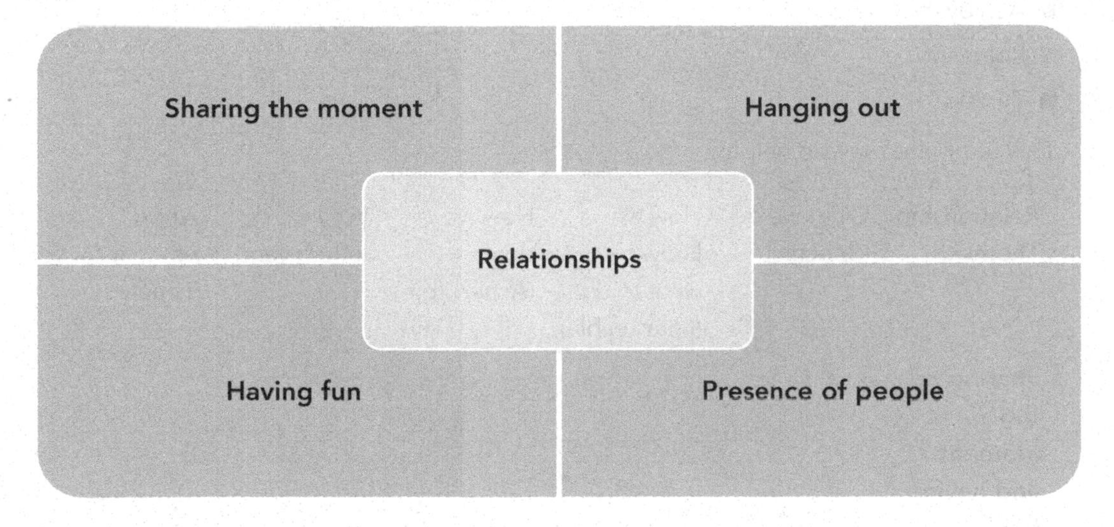

Group Activity

Consider the following questions (these can apply in most settings):

- In the classroom, where does the curriculum emphasise the opportunity for development of relationships?
- During the school day, where do the opportunities for 'just hanging out & having fun' happen?
- As a team, do you actively create opportunities for relational interactions just by your presence?

As a team, identify where these areas need to be developed and write an action plan. These should be based on SMART objectives.

- Specific.
- Measurable.
- Achievable.
- Relevant.
- Timely.

This template may be helpful:

Relationship Themes:	What we do (Specific)	How we know what to do (Measurable)	How we do it (Achievable)	Why we do it (Relevant)	When we do it (Timely)
Sharing the moment and having fun					

Material well-being

The United Nations Convention on the Rights of Persons with Disability (UNCRPD) recognises the right of people with an intellectual disability to live in a place of their choosing and with people of their choice (Article 19) (United Nations, 2006). The links between environmental factors such as living conditions and social

Enabling Capable Environments © Pavilion Publishing and Media Ltd and its licensors 2024.

attitudes can have a significant impact on people's social inclusion and participation (Emerson & Hatton, 2014). It is also recognised that, where people live and who they spend their time with, does have an overall impact on their well-being and quality of life. In our clinical experience, people with an intellectual disability do not always have a say in where they live or who they live with. The lack of opportunity for paid work also has an impact on the choices people have about where they live and where they spend their time. Research by Conder & Mirfin-Veitch (2020) describes how a training project for people with an intellectual disability on money matters was positively received by people who attended, expanding their knowledge and skills in managing a budget. They discuss that such initiatives are rare, and that wider community support should have more of a focus on developing and supporting opportunities for financial and material well-being.

Later work by Carlsson & Adolfsson (2022) interviewed people with an intellectual disability living in the community about their perspectives on their living conditions. While all reported that they would choose to live in their own home and recognised the need for support to do this, their experience was that dependence on support in daily life 'infringed' on their sense of adult social status and control of their life. Examples of such infringements include staff using rooms in the house to hold meetings (that did not include the individual) lack of access to phones or internet to call family, and not having privacy when family came to visit. This study illustrates the need for support to be focused on people's well-being, community participation and maintaining friends and relationships, and to understand how support can become a barrier in these areas. The challenge for us as support providers is to consider how we are a catalyst for enhancing people's well-being rather than inhibiting it.

Personal development

'Personal development' will mean different things to different people, but it typically involves the development of personal skills and educational opportunities to reflect people's goals and aspirations. It is essential to recognise that this applies across the lifespan, not just something that is considered for younger people (Schalock & Alonso, 2015).

Research has shown that adults with an intellectual disability often do not routinely have opportunities to develop new skills or pursue interests (Bigby & Beadle-Brown, 2016). The Care Quality Commission (CQC, 2022) promotes a social model of disability that they recommend should:

- Offer a range of learning opportunities for people as part of a lifelong learning approach.
- Ensure people can develop skills to support community participation.
- Promote recreational and leisure activities that reflect people's needs and interests.
- Ensure there are opportunities to develop a wide range of personal and social relationships.
- Follow a lifestyle of their choosing, including their social life.

One way of doing this is to ensure that each person using the service has a pathway for personal development based on assessing their needs and aspirations (this can be based on a Person-Centred Plan (PCP) (Sanderson, 2000). PCP can promote a co-produced approach to service planning where people are more involved in the design and delivery of services to better meet their needs. Having a strengths-based approach builds on people's existing personal resources to work out their personal development goals and means of achieving them.

Physical well-being

Although recent efforts have been made to address health inequities, people with an intellectual disability can experience difficulties in accessing high-quality care (World Health Organisation: WHO, 2020).

The barriers that people with an intellectual disability face when trying to get equal access to health care are also well documented. Examples include:

- Their communication needs are not being met.
- Lack of services.
- Lack of training for health professionals.
- Lack of training for social care/education staff.

Our understanding of physical health is broader than just being based on the absence of illness; it needs to include an understanding of how other broader factors influence health. For people with intellectual disabilities, there can be specific factors impacting their physical health such as being at a higher risk of certain health conditions linked to their diagnosis. For example, people with a diagnosis of Cornelia de Lange syndrome may be more likely to have reflux or Gastroesophageal Reflux Disease (GERD). Other individual factors include not having the means to communicate their health symptoms, which can result in a decline in health

Enabling Capable Environments © Pavilion Publishing and Media Ltd and its licensors 2024.

being missed or incorrectly linked to the person's intellectual disability. Such misconceptions about people's health needs lead to significant repercussions, and people have died because of constipation, choking, issues relating to diabetes, pneumonia, or other respiratory issues. These illnesses are recognised as preventable, but they lead to people with an intellectual disability dying on average 20 years younger than the general population (O'Leary *et al.*, 2018).

Most of these issues can and should be addressed with detailed health action planning, but research and reports show that there are gaps in such planning due in some part to those providing support not having support or training to develop such plans. Such gaps in knowledge and skills can lead to:

- People living in services that do not promote physical activity, resulting in people living sedentary lives.
- Poor nutrition, in part because of being reliant on others to support nutritional needs.
- Polypharmacy, where people are prescribed multiple medications with limited consideration to how these interact with each other and impact upon health and well-being in the longer term.
- Limited opportunities and resources to pursue recreational and leisure activities.
- Those who support the person not understanding the need for or supporting access to regular health assessments.
- Routine health screening is not made accessible, or there is a lack of reasonable adjustment to access these.

Recommendations to address such health disparities should include:

- Better health promotion programmes focused on addressing the specific needs of people with an intellectual disability.
- Better understanding of why people with an intellectual disability do not get access to better support for their health needs.
- Identifying what training and skills direct support staff need to promote access to support for health needs.
- A better understanding of the social determinants of health for people with an intellectual disability, for example, their reliance on others for support to access healthcare and a lack of reasonable adjustments being significant factors in poorer outcomes.

The shift towards person-centred care or patient-centred care is internationally recognised. The World Health Organization has committed to creating a framework for putting people at the centre of healthcare, people-centred health services which are described as:

> *'...an approach to care that consciously adopts the perspectives of individuals, families, and communities, and sees them as participants as well as beneficiaries of trusted health systems that respond to their needs and preferences in humane and holistic ways. People-centred care requires that people have the education and support they need to make decisions and participate in their own care. It is organised around the health needs and expectations of people rather than diseases.'* (WHO, 2016, p2)

There is a requirement for a more systemic approach to meeting the healthcare needs of people with an intellectual disability, which requires policymakers to think innovatively and provide funding to support such initiatives. What is clear is that we do not need more reports repeating the same narrative about how and why people with an intellectual disability are facing such health inequalities and risk dying 20 years younger than their peers. We need action policies based on the recommendations from such reports.

Self-determination

The importance of self-determination for people with an intellectual disability was first discussed in 1972 by Nirje, who discussed the need for people with an intellectual disability to live life and 'experience self-determination'. This discussion was against the backdrop of the movement to deinstitutionalise services.

However, many of the environments that people with an intellectual disability continue to access or live in are congregate settings, which are a barrier to people having choice and control in their lives (the very essence of self-determination). Some research has shown that, beyond the activities of day-to-day living, people with an intellectual disability have limited opportunities to exercise choice and control in their lives (Bigby & Beadle-Brown, 2016). Other research has identified that people moving from restrictive to community-based settings were more likely to have enhanced opportunities for choice and control (Stancliffe *et al.*, 2020).

However, we should be very cautious before assuming that a physical environment alone is an influence or the only variable of self-determination. Self-determination needs to be considered within the context of where people are and who is around

 Enabling Capable Environments © Pavilion Publishing and Media Ltd and its licensors 2024.

them. This context includes more than the immediate environment; it considers the barriers to self-determination and what will act as enablers.

In 2015, Schalock & Verdugo identified that self-determination should be part of how services are delivered; services should ensure that people can decide and make things happen in their own lives rather than these actions being imposed on them or decided for them. They state that:

'Self-determined action is goal-oriented, driven by preferences and interests, and ultimately serves to enable people to enhance the quality of their lives.'

Wehmeyer (2020) adds that being self-determined, 'that is, making things happen in one's life', has been linked to multiple positive outcomes, including enhanced quality of life and life satisfaction.

People need self-determination skills, for example, the skills and the opportunity to make choices. These skills do not appear by chance just because of the physical environment; this can help, but it is insufficient. Those in supporting roles need skills and mentorship in advancing opportunities for people to exercise self-determination. However, equally, people with an intellectual disability need the opportunity to learn these skills (for more details on this, see Chapter 7 and Chapter 8).

Thinking space

The opportunities to have choice and control are very much influenced by the context of where people are and who is around them. Organisations must ensure that their mission and values are explicit about their pursuit of self-determination. For example:

- Are people in support/education roles aspirational about the individual's right to make choices and determine their goals and aspirations irrespective of the level of intellectual disability?
- Do people ensure that support for decision-making is maximised for people, for example communication support?
- Are the systems and processes within the organisation aligned to the individual's wishes and needs, for example the use of person-centred planning tools?
- Do support plans reflect the aspirations and needs of the individual and explicitly direct staff on how to provide support to meet these?

Consider each of these four questions either for an organisation you work in or one that you access for support and note examples of good practices and areas for development.

Social inclusion

Schalock & Alonso (2015), in their discussion on social inclusion, refer to people with an intellectual disability experiencing community integration and having the right support to have a role they value in their community. However, research shows that people with an intellectual disability are more likely to have a smaller social network and experience a higher rate of loneliness than others (Mithen *et al*., 2015). More recent research by Emerson *et al*., (2021) found that people with an intellectual disability reported high levels of loneliness (51%) and experienced limited social connections within their community and that this low level of social connections had a negative impact on their overall well-being.

This suggests that more than just being present in a community setting is needed to support inclusion. What is needed is a more systematic approach to people's circles of support and a drive to ensure these are robust and not left to chance. For people with an intellectual disability, their circle of support can look very different to ours. For example, the people who are part of the day-to-day lives of adults with an intellectual disability may be people who are in paid roles, and the places people with an intellectual disability go to may be placed in a community setting but are

Enabling Capable Environments © Pavilion Publishing and Media Ltd and its licensors 2024.

not for all members of the community. We are not suggesting that specific settings for people with an intellectual disability are not needed; many are, but if this is the only experience people with an intellectual disability have of community-based settings, then they are less likely to have the opportunity to meet new friends and to be part of their community at a broader level.

Circle of support

For many of us, our circle of support will look like the circle in Figure 1.2:

Figure 1.2: Circle of support

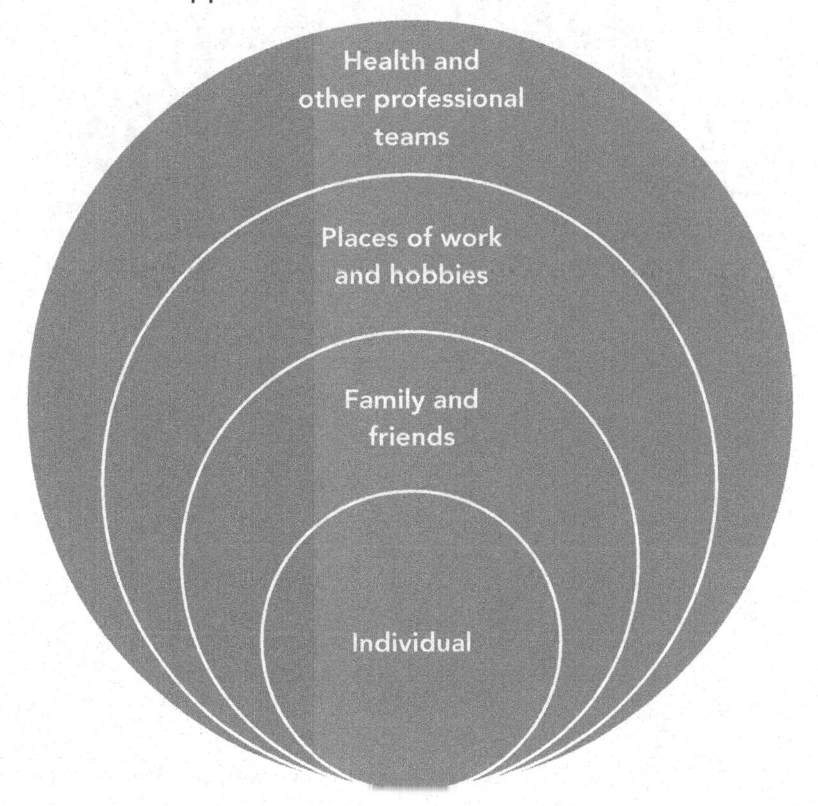

Enabling Capable Environments © Pavilion Publishing and Media Ltd and its licensors 2024.

Thinking space

For many of us, our day-to-day experiences are marked by a social support network of family and friends and time spent in places that hold meaning and enjoyment for us.

Consider the person you are supporting. Does their circle of support look different to this and what may need to change in their circle to reflect a circle of meaningful support to them? Use the circle below to do this:

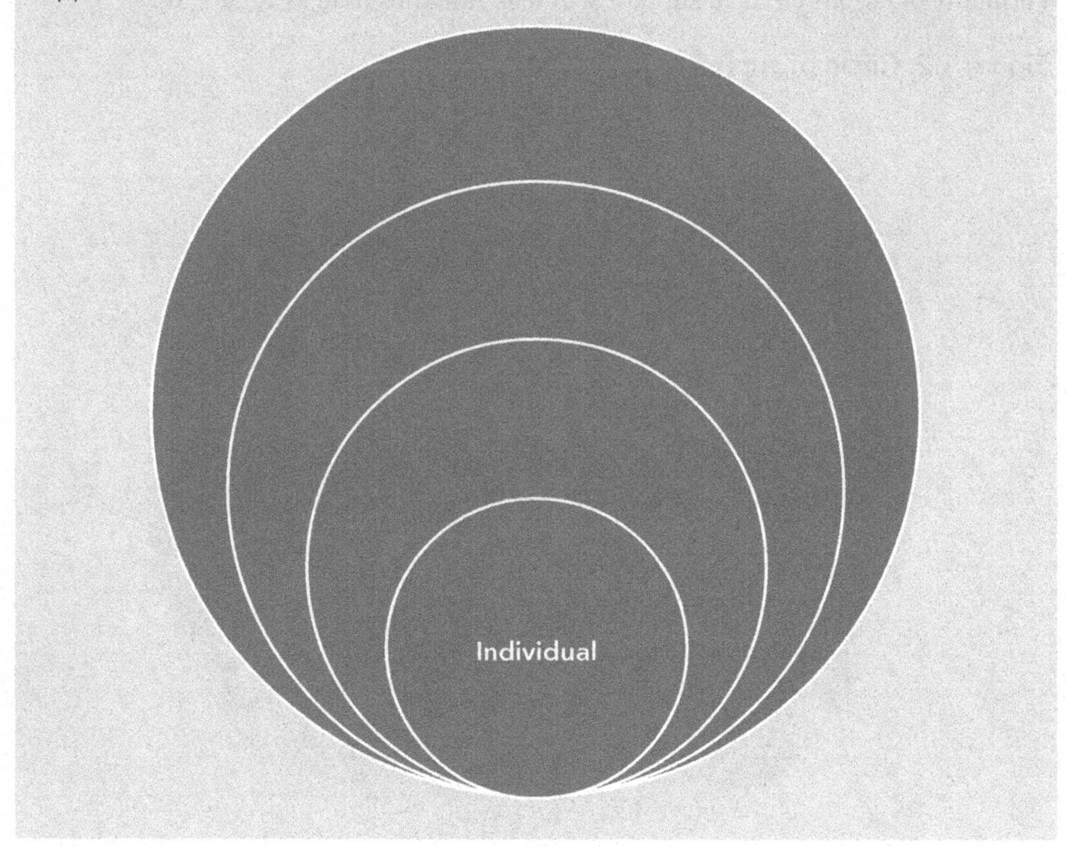

Rights

A human right is an entitlement that belongs to every person, regardless of whether they have an intellectual disability or not. The Human Rights Act (1998) applies to every person in the UK.

The Human Rights Act places a duty on public authorities to ensure that all actions and decisions that they make take these rights into account. If a public authority

Enabling Capable Environments © Pavilion Publishing and Media Ltd and its licensors 2024.

does not, it may be in breach of an individual's human rights, and they could be taken to court.

Article 3 – freedom from torture and inhuman or degrading treatment – is a very important right for people with learning disabilities. People with learning disabilities have the right to receive care and support that is dignified and respectful. A public authority must intervene if a person deliberately inflicts mental or physical harm on a person with a learning disability, which includes physical and/or psychological abuse in a health or care setting. The state has a duty to protect people from such treatment and investigate allegations.

Article 8 – a right to respect for private and family life – is also a very important right. People with learning disabilities have a right to live their lives privately, to enjoy family relationships (including the right to live with their own family), and to enjoy their homes peacefully without interference from public authorities.

Article 12 – the right to marry – means that people with learning disabilities have the right to marry and to start a family, just like everybody else.

Article 14 – protection from discrimination – requires all rights and freedoms set out in the Act to be applied without discrimination (direct or indirect). In other words, people with learning disabilities should not be stopped from enjoying any of the other rights in the Act because of their disability.

The British Institute of Human Rights (BIHR: 2016) has produced a booklet explaining how each of these rights applies to what practitioners need to do to ensure they uphold these rights. The booklet is available at:

https://knowyourhumanrights.co.uk/resources/BIHR_Mental_Health_Practitioner_Resource_LearningDisability.pdf

We would recommend support teams use the booklet as part of training, reflective supervision, team meetings, etc. as a way of ensuring the rights of people with an intellectual disability remain at the forefront of their practice.

Person-centred approaches in the support of person-centred actions

Person-Centred Planning (PCP) is a core feature of national guidance and policies (Department of Health, 2012; National Institute for Health and Care Excellence,

Enabling Capable Environments © Pavilion Publishing and Media Ltd and its licensors 2024.

NICE: 2015). It was first outlined by O'Brien & O'Brien (2002) within the context of the conceptual framework of inclusion. The aim was to develop individualised support through a planning process focused on an individual's preferences and strengths. There are several formats for person-centred planning such as Person Futures Planning (Sanderson, 2000); Planning Alternative Tomorrows with Hope (PATH) (O'Brien *et al.*, 2010) and Making Action Plans (MAPS) (O'Brien *et al.*, 2010).

Sanderson (2000) describes five critical features of PCP:

- The person is at the centre of the plan.
- Family members and friends are the key partners in planning.
- A PCP reflects what is important to the individual, their preferences and what support is needed to reflect these.
- The plan results in actions that are about their life and reflect what is possible and not what is available.
- The plan results in ongoing development. Person-centred planning intends to move the focus from what a service can offer to the individual, to tailoring services to the individual and their family's preferences and needs.

However, limitations to the applications of PCP in practice have been identified. Ratti *et al.*'s (2016) systemic review of the literature recognised that, overall, the empirical evidence to support the effectiveness of PCP had a moderate impact on some outcomes for individuals such as community participation, engagement in activities and choice-making.

Previously Mansell & Beadle-Brown's (2004) review of person-centred planning recognised that it can become limited to the development of a plan, which is not then applied in practice. They discuss that person-centred action is needed. They outline examples of how to translate a PCP into person-centred action. Staff training should be focused on facilitating change. The focus of supervision should be on change for the individual.

Other person-centred approaches include Person-Centred Active Support and Positive Behaviour Support. Both are discussed in more detail in Chapter 7 and Chapter 9.

Enabling Capable Environments © Pavilion Publishing and Media Ltd and its licensors 2024.

Conclusion

We have established in this chapter that the application of the **quality-of-life** concept establishes the need for individualised support based on the principles of human rights, inclusion, equity and self-determination. However, in daily practice, these domains need to be translated into tangible **person-centred actions**. We have identified that just being aware of these quality-of-life concepts is insufficient as, without a clear vision and systems of support, services and teams can struggle to apply them in their daily practice.

- Having a clear vision and a shared philosophy based on these quality-of-life domains can help shape clear leadership roles which in turn support the necessary activities of support staff to ensure better quality-of-life outcomes for individuals.
- Such leadership roles need to incorporate the principles of **practice leadership** where the focus is to support the application of these principles in day-to-day practices.
- Services need to be organised in a way that **enables capable environments** to ensure positive outcomes about participation, well-being, and inclusion (PCAS, PCP & PBS).
- Finally, the standards and outcomes of **Periodic Service Reviews (PSRs)** are co-produced to reflect the dynamic roles people have in ensuring that quality of life is the central tenet of service design, delivery, and evaluation. In this book, we present a more **unified framework** of support (Figure 1.3) that moves beyond just an ecological perspective but considers a more holistic humanistic understanding of people's life goals and builds systems of support.

This chapter sets the scene for the remainder of this book. We believe there needs to be a more unified approach to models of support (Figure 1.3) for people with an intellectual disability and for those who support them in whatever setting or capacity.

Figure 1.3: A unified approach to person-centred supports

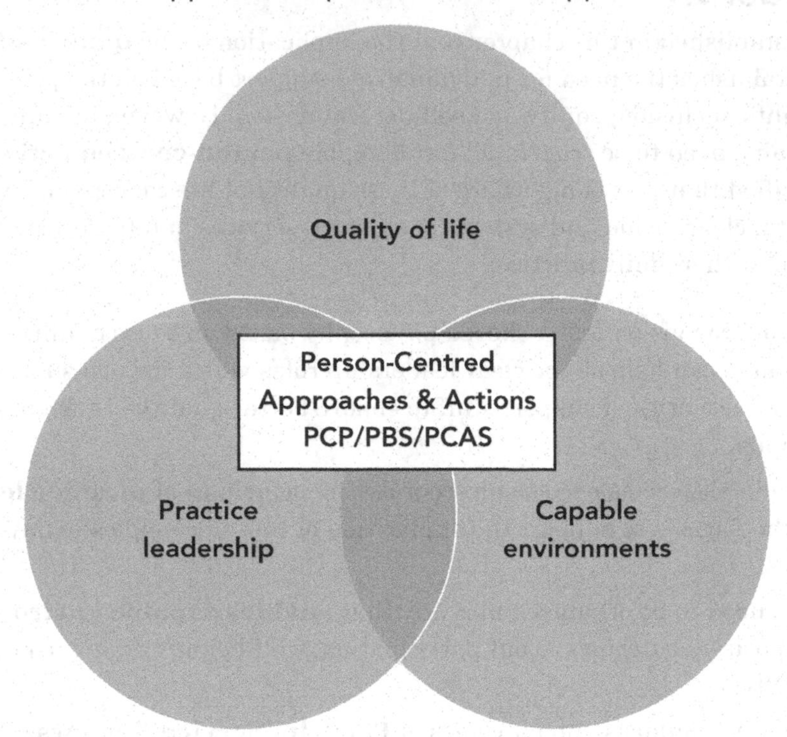

Enabling Capable Environments © Pavilion Publishing and Media Ltd and its licensors 2024.

Chapter 2: Enabling capable environments

'Our job is not to fix people, but to design effective environments'
(Rob Horner, Royal College of Psychiatrists, 2007)

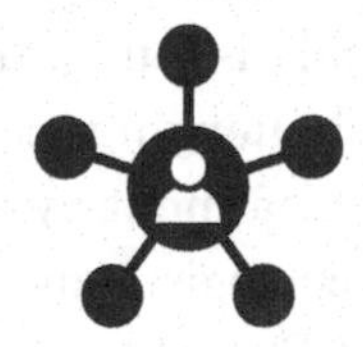

Chapter contents:

- What are capable environments?
- Understanding of the links between behaviour and the environment.
- Identifying the characteristics of a capable environment.
- Appraising capable environments.
- Enabling capable environments.
- Positive outcomes.
- Paving a way to success.

Learning outcomes

After reading this chapter and completing the suggested activities and reflection, the reader should be able to:

- Identify the characteristics of what a capable environment is in their practice/home/school setting.
- Develop and appraise the characteristics in their setting.
- Demonstrate the principles of co-production in the appraisal and implementation of a capable environments Periodic Service Review (PSR).

Enabling Capable Environments © Pavilion Publishing and Media Ltd and its licensors 2024.

Introduction

This is the first of three chapters within this book to explore capable environments as a framework of support. In this first chapter, we provide an overview of what the characteristics of a capable environment are and then provide some detailed examples of how to enable these into practice. There are subsequent chapters which outline how to embed and sustain a capable environment framework (Chapters 3 and 4).

There has been a change in our understanding of what impacts the quality of life of individuals with an intellectual disability. In the past, and still common even now, behaviours described as challenging have been regarded as a problem within the individual that requires treatment by allied health professionals such as behavioural specialists, psychologists and psychiatrists (Royal College of Psychiatrists *et al*., 2007). This RCP report and more recent research now understands that creating environments that better meet people's needs and provide access to meaningful activities that focus on well-being will more likely see a reduction in 'challenging behaviour' by enhancing people's quality of life. This understanding has led to considerable research into and advances in practices that increase the quality of service delivery and thereby increase the quality of life of individuals with an intellectual disability (Schalock, 2004).

In 1994, Emerson *et al* identified that services designed for people with intellectual disabilities were commonly institutions or hospital environments. There began to be an understanding that these environments were negatively impacting the individuals who were living there (Emerson *et al*., 1994). McGill and Toogood (1994) showed that these environments had some common features that made them unsuitable for offering a good quality of life for those being supported. For example, some of these environments had:

- A lack of choice and control.
- Practices that were abusive which in turn created fear and distress for the people in the service.
- Limited contact between staff and the people being supported, therefore increasing people's isolation and segregation
- Limited opportunities, for example, having interesting things to do, spending time with people that like you.
- Limited access to preferred items (or, in fact, any items, due to locked cupboards and doors, etc.).

 Enabling Capable Environments © Pavilion Publishing and Media Ltd and its licensors 2024.

These environments could lead to the person using their behaviour to indicate, in whatever way they can, that they wanted to avoid things they don't like, seek interaction or connection with people, indicate they have no choices or control over their lives (more details about functions and messages of behaviour can be found in chapter 9). The key message here is that we now know that such institutional settings and practices are very likely to be a setting event (making something more likely to happen) for the likelihood that behaviour that challenges will occur. This is due to these environments not meeting the person's needs, causing distress and becoming a challenge for them.

It became clear at this time that there was a need to move away from these institutionalised environments and focus more on people living in their own homes in the community. Although it was not recognised at the time, it was not enough to simply move current supports into community settings. Instead, an essential shift had to be made to challenge these institutional practices that hindered quality of life. McGill & Toogood (1994) discussed 'providing helpful environments' that were structured to increase choice, engagement in meaningful activity and interactions, and enhance skills with a person-centred focus. Over the years, this has been discussed and expanded upon (Royal College of Psychiatrists, 2007), leading to the development of the capable environment's framework in 2014 and its update in 2020 (McGill *et al.*, 2014; McGill *et al.*, 2020).

'Capable environments' are a systematic, theoretically driven approach that is focused on the quality of support design and support provision for people with an intellectual disability. McGill (2014 & 2020) outlines the 12 characteristics that can support capable environments:

> *'These characteristics share two defining features. First, they produce positive outcomes for individuals and their supporters such as enhanced quality of life. Second, they prevent many instances of challenging behaviour'* (p3).

Hume *et al* (2021) demonstrated that the use of such a framework as an intervention helps staff provide effective personalised support, a foundation for positive behaviour support (PBS), and other personalised supports outlined throughout this book.

Understanding behaviour in the context of the environment

Carr *et al*. (1999) identified that a "key aim of positive behaviour support is to address two kinds of deficits, one being environmental deficiencies such as lack of, choice, engagement, and organisation within the settings; the second is presented as behaviour repertoire deficiencies such as barriers to communication or social skills". Behaviours that challenge are more likely to occur in disorganised environments, those that fail to promote quality of life outcomes, and those that are unresponsive to personal needs. Therefore, addressing such 'environmental deficits' by ensuring environments are more capable would be a rational foundation for support design irrespective of the presence of behaviours described as challenging and, more importantly, ensuring our attention is focused on environmental (ecological) strategies that smooth the fit between the person and their environment (Donnellan *et al*., 1988).

The second deficit that Carr *et al*. (1999) refer to is around a lack of communication and social skills, where people with an intellectual disability are not supported or respected in their decisions or are not provided with the opportunity to learn skills to meet their own needs. For example, getting to do what they want, when they want, and with whom, and avoiding what they don't like and that includes people they don't like!

In summary, this failure to meet a person's needs can result in behaviours that challenge. There are many ways that people's environments and lack of opportunity to exercise choice and control can impact how people may behave, but in general, there are some broad categories that may help point support teams in the direction of understanding why behaviours that challenge occur.

Traditionally, it has been acknowledged that four broad categories help in understanding why a person may be engaging in behaviours that challenge. These are:

- To escape/avoid difficult situations.
- To indicate a need for access to social attention/interaction.
- To meet a sensory need that helps them.
- To gain access to a tangible item they need or want.

(Chapter 9 provides more detail on these categories.)

Enabling Capable Environments © Pavilion Publishing and Media Ltd and its licensors 2024.

As discussed earlier, services and supports designed for people with an intellectual disability have some common features that increase the likelihood of behaviours that challenge. These common features lead to:

- People seeking to escape and avoid distressing situations. This may be due to environments not meeting personal or sensory needs, communication not being tailored to the person's needs resulting in confusion, tasks or activities that the person doesn't enjoy being mandatory, etc.
- People seeking out contact from others due to a lack of interaction from others, low staffing levels, expectations for tasks to be completed over building relationships and engaging in meaningful, others being unsure or unwilling to interact, etc.
- People seeking stimulation due to environments lacking varied activities, interaction, or feedback.
- People seeking access to preferred items due to access being limited.

As it is common for individuals with an intellectual disability to also have communication support needs, it is understandable that, in environments such as those described above, challenging behaviour may be likely to be the only way for the individual to communicate their needs or be an indicator of unmet needs (Emerson *et al.*, 1994). It may be that services in themselves work as 'establishing operations' or setting events (more detail in Chapter 9) for behaviours that challenge. In other words, environments that are developed to support individuals with an intellectual disability instead may provide an environment that increases the likelihood that challenging behaviour may occur (Emerson *et al.*, 1994).

When behaviours that challenge do occur, there has been and continues to be a focus on the individual and the interventions needed to fix or treat the 'problem behaviour' (McGill *et al.*, 2020), but creating environments that help meet the person's needs is a more effective way of making a sustainable change. A capable environment can be defined as an environment associated with reduced frequency and/or severity of behaviour that challenges (McGill *et al.*, 2020). Studies show that 'many of the environments where individuals at risk of displaying challenging behaviour are supported are not nearly as capable as they could be' (McGill *et al.*, 2014). Emerson *et al.* (1994) suggest that these environments should be the opposite of the unhelpful environments discussed above and should provide access to preferred items, access to social contact, and access to meaningful activities and interactions. Capable environments help

Enabling Capable Environments © Pavilion Publishing and Media Ltd and its licensors 2024.

move the focus away from the disputed notion that problems reside with and within an individual, towards changing the challenging environments around the person. In addition, these capable environments should be part of all support models irrespective of challenging behaviour.

The characteristics of capable environments

A Capable Environment is comprised of 12 characteristics. Each characteristic, when met, is known to be associated with an increased quality of life for people with an intellectual disability (see Chapters 3 and 4). Each characteristic is supported by an evidence base demonstrating its association with increases in quality of life and therefore a reduction in the environmental contributors that may lead to behaviours described as challenging. Further, some evidence suggests that implementation of the capable environment's framework can lead to a reduction in the occurrence and severity of behaviour that challenges.

Enabling Capable Environments © Pavilion Publishing and Media Ltd and its licensors 2024.

Figure 2.1: The characteristics of a capable environments framework

Mindful, Skilled Carers
Acceptable Physical Environment
Communication
Engagement in Meaningful Activity
Positive Social Interaction
Consistent and Predictable Environments
The Person
Personal Care and Health Support
Relationships with Family and Friends
Independent Functioning
Opportunities for Choice
Effective Management and Support
Effective Organisational Context

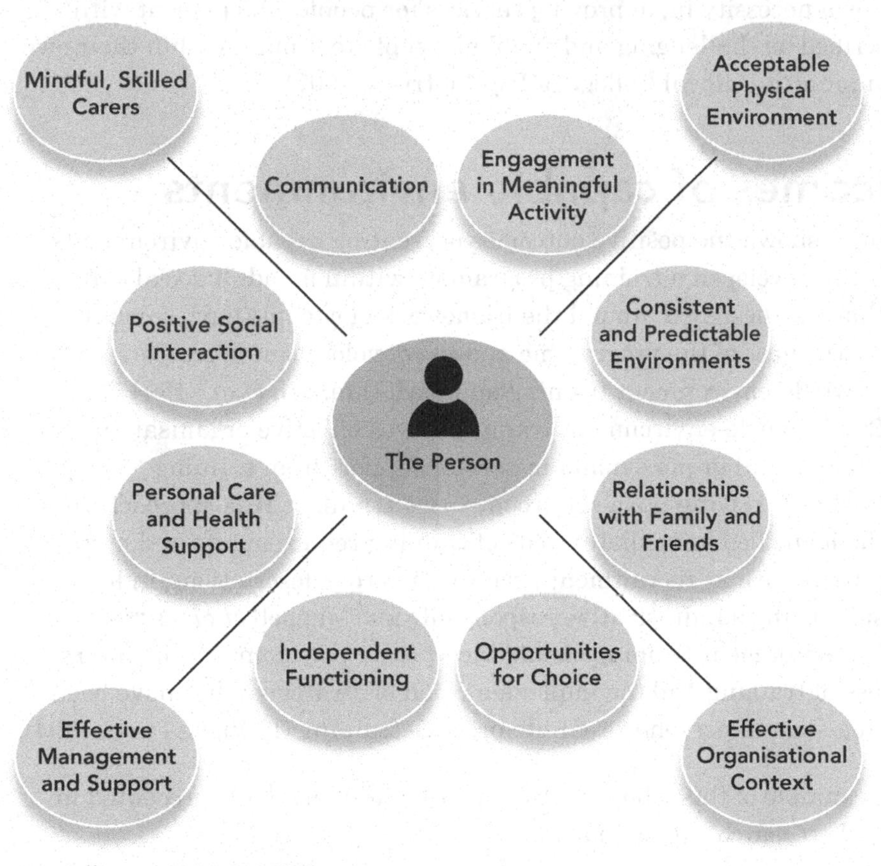

(McGill *et al* 2014 & 2020)

Figure 2.1 shows the capable environments framework. The inner eight characteristics focus on the direct support for the individual (see Chapter 3) and the outer four characteristics concentrate on what surrounds the person and the systems of support that are in place (see Chapter 4).

The benefits of capable environments

There are several proposed positive outcomes of capable environments, for example, McGill *et al*. (2020) say that:

> *'Such an approach promises substantial quality of life improvements for individuals, better work environments for staff and a reduction in the costs associated with specialist care and out-of-area placements.'* (p1)

The Royal College of Psychiatrists also published guidance which cites capable environments as a necessity in, improving services for people who present with behaviour described as challenging and enabling people to remain within their own homes and communities (Royal College of Psychiatrists, 2007).

The outcomes of capable environments

Research has also shown the positive outcomes of creating capable environments. Hume *et al*. (2021) developed a training programme within an adult social care organisation that was designed around the framework of capable environments. Vital to the effectiveness of the programme and the development of support planning was a whole-environment training approach (Mansell *et al*., 1994 & McGill *et al*., 2020). Whole-environment training drives effective organisational change, through practical in-person and in-service support from training facilitators, not simply relying upon classroom-based training. This approach goes further than the identified immediate needs of training requirements and may focus on other areas such as recruitment practices, job role descriptions, induction training and supporting administrative responsibilities (Mansell *et al*., 1994). This model of whole environment training should incorporate a system that monitors the effectiveness of training and the implementation of strategies that have been developed during such in-person/in-real-life practice training (LaVigna *et al*., 1994).

A more recent example of this whole environment training model is presented in Hume *et al* (2021) research, which found:

- An **increase in engagement in meaningful activity** using the Active Support Measure (ASM) (Mansell *et al*., 2005) and Momentary Time Sampling (MTS). Active Support is a model of support for people with an intellectual disability that enhances relationships and increases engagement in meaningful activity (Mansell & Beadle-Brown, 2012). The ASM is a tool that measures the level of active staff support provided.
- The level of **staff interaction, staff assistance, and praise increasing**.
- A **decrease in the frequency and episodic severity** of behavioural incidents.
- A **reduction in the use of as-required emergency medication** for 'managing behaviour' (As-required medication is a medication that is taken when and if needed).

 Enabling Capable Environments © Pavilion Publishing and Media Ltd and its licensors 2024.

Thinking space

You may think that these 12 characteristics require little support to facilitate and may occur naturally, but McGill *et al.* (1994) show these "helpful environments" do not ordinarily occur in services without structured support and systematic implementation. On the contrary, naturally occurring day-to-day events are more likely to lead to unhelpful environments. Therefore, it is important to consider how to develop and support a capable environment.

Below, we detail how capable environments have been developed, implemented, and supported to increase the quality of life of people with intellectual disabilities and, as a side effect, to reduce behaviours that challenge. Throughout this case study we also provide useful resources that will allow the reader to replicate this process and create capable environments within their own homes, classrooms, or services.

Appraising and implementing capable environments

Case study

The capable environments framework was at the centre of the work conducted by Hume *et al.* (2021), who utilised it to appraise, plan, monitor, and evaluate current support and constructively identify opportunities for development. The authors supported managers in assessing their services, alongside their staff teams, using a modified version of McGill *et al.*'s (2020) characteristics of capable environments table, called the Capable Environments Appraisal (CEA) (see Appendix One: Capable Environments Appraisal). Amendments to the original table include replacing the 'illustrative evidence' column with two blank columns that appraisers complete with their staff teams based on knowledge of and observations within their services. The decision to adapt the characteristics of the capable environments table and to use it as an appraisal tool in such a way was inspired by the structure within the United Response 'What does good look like' checklist (Beadle-Brown & Murphy, 2016) and the PSR format (LaVigna *et al.*, 1994) which focused on opportunities for development, rather than focusing on 'problems'. These columns supported the appraisers to consider both what was going well in their services, related to the specific characteristics, and to identify opportunities for development and improvement.

An example of a completed section on the Capable Environments Appraisal (CEA) is shown in Table 2.1.

Enabling Capable Environments © Pavilion Publishing and Media Ltd and its licensors 2024.

Table 2.1: Example of a Capable Environments Appraisal for one component				
Characteristic	What does this involve?	Why is this important?	Evidence	
			Working well (what works for Sandra)	*Opportunities for development (What we need to do to make it better)*
Support for participation in meaningful activity.	Carers provide tailored assistance for the individual to engage meaningfully in preferred domestic, leisure, work activities and social interactions. Assistance/ support meaningfully employs speech, manual signs, symbols or objects of reference as appropriate.	Challenging behaviour is less likely when the person is meaningfully occupied. Skilled support ensures that individuals can participate at least partially even in relatively complex activities so that they experience success and can work through difficult tasks knowing that have the support they need. This can also help the person to cope with demands and difficulties that may have given rise to challenging behaviour but are avoided due a positive and supportive expertise. Most people (with and without an intellectual disability) like to be busy.	*On a few occasions, Sandra is seen participating in the upkeep of her garden. *Sandra is supported to engage in some domestic tasks (folding laundry, mopping and occasional dusting) within her home using graded assistance. *Visual symbols are used to support an understanding of the order of tasks. Sandra has a variety of meals and snacks but are all prepared by the staff team.	Support to engage in gardening should be more consistently implemented every day. Time spent in community setting engaging in activities selected by Sandra need to frequently occur. Sandra should have the time and opportunity to plan her day each morning deciding on what activities should happen and when. A plan for Sandra should be developed around how to enhance and maintain her home environment

Enabling Capable Environments © Pavilion Publishing and Media Ltd and its licensors 2024.

			**Narrative from the authors: While the experiences in this column may be important, they reflect a mundane experience which is lacking interesting and motivating life experiences. We need to look at opportunities to expand Sandra's life experience in a way that has more meaning and value to her. **	Sandra will plan her meals and be supported to learn how to prepare snacks and how to plan and prepare a meal for her family. Support staff should use positive language or an upbeat style when supporting Sandra.

This is just one example of one section of the Capable Environments Appraisal tool. Those utilising the tool will need to complete each section of the appraisal (Appendix Number One).

Implementing capable environments

Introducing the appraisal

Before enabling an environment to be more capable, it is important to understand what is currently working in that environment and where there are opportunities to develop. Using the capable environments appraisal tool is an effective way of understanding the current environment and its needs.

Before conducting an appraisal of the environment, it is important to consider how to complete this assessment and the impact it may have. Staff at all levels must understand that this is a collaborative process and that they will be fully listened to and included throughout. It must be made clear that they will be an integral part of identifying strengths, identifying opportunities, and developing support to make changes where agreed.

Thinking space

Think of a time when your practice was being assessed/appraised. This may have been for a university presentation, your driving test, or your manager assessing your practice at work.

How did this feel?

What helped ease your worries?

What helped make the process better?

It's important to think about the staff and the management team's experiences of being appraised. Staff at all levels have likely had several experiences of being assessed that may not always have been positive. It's possible their experiences of being assessed may be associated with feelings of criticism and as a process that was done *to them*, not *with them*. It may be that staff and managers are used to appraisals only highlighting things that are not being done well. This could lead to an understandable lack of willingness to participate or resistance to the process. When completing a capable environment appraisal, frame the process positively and ensure everyone has a voice at each stage. This can be achieved through:

- Communicating clearly that the appraisal will focus on both achievements as well as areas that can be enhanced.
- Express that a good life for the person being supported doesn't simply happen, it needs to be planned for and everyone needs to plan this together.
- Explain that the process is not a way to admonish the team or the service. It is a self-reflection and strengths-based process.
- Stress that the process is collaborative and something that is being done together. No decisions will be made at any stage without coming together.
- Discuss the process involving all levels of staff.
- Reassure teams that the appraisal process will require spending time together in practice to hear their views and gain their vital perspectives.
- Explain that this looks to identify areas of good practice and opportunities for development and that this will be done together.
- Communicate that understanding where the service currently is will help to enhance this in the future. This will be completed in partnership with support from the appraiser.

Enabling Capable Environments © Pavilion Publishing and Media Ltd and its licensors 2024.

- Being mindful of language is also key. It is best to stay away from language such as 'inspection' or 'audit' and use terms such as 'appraisal'. Staff may have previous experiences of being audited and inspected and this may not have been a positive or collaborative process. This could skew people's perceptions of this process.
- Offer opportunities for people to raise concerns and equally share exemplars of good practice or ideas that will enhance the quality of support.
- Allow teams to consider what has been shared and provide contact details, as well as ensuring time is scheduled for any follow-up questions.

Thinking space

Take time to think about how you will introduce the appraisal within a classroom or service.

1. Who might you need to speak to before you introduce the appraisal?
2. How will you introduce the appraisal? A team meeting with everyone? Small group discussions? One-to-one sessions?
3. How will you explain the capable environments appraisal to your team, ensuring they are aware it is a way to better meet and organise a person's support?
4. How will you ensure the messages above are clearly communicated?
5. How will you reassure people who are nervous about being observed?
6. How will you ensure everyone's voice is heard at all stages of the process?

Completing the appraisal

Only after introducing capable environments and the appraisal process, should you conduct the appraisal. This should be agreed upon collectively after time has been spent together in services, meeting with staff to understand their perspectives, achievements and concerns, as well as observing practice.

Before conducting the appraisal, the appraisor(s) must understand the CEA and consider the types of areas they should be focusing on when completing each section. In Hume *et al.* (2021), appraisers were trainees who were being supported to become practice leaders within their services. Each trainee was undertaking a programme to build capable environments through practice leadership, delivered by positive behaviour support specialists. They were frontline managers who spent time in their services working alongside staff teams regularly and were asked to select one focus person to concentrate on during their meetings and observations. Based on the environment you work in; consider who is in the best position to take on this role and who would have the most influence on change. We strongly recommend that appraisers include someone from the service, school, or health setting and not a solely external individual. This model focuses on working in collaboration and recognises the expertise within the service/family/education setting.

Below is a list of questions the appraisers should ask themselves while meeting with teams, conducting observations, and completing the CEA.

Table 2.2: Capable environments areas of focus

Characteristic	Areas of focus
Positive social interactions	Appraisers should be looking for the types of interactions that the person with an intellectual disability experiences throughout the day and across all of those who work with them (education staff/ family members etc). ■ When the person looks at those that support them or come close to them, do the staff members reciprocate this and start a conversation/ask them if they would like to do something/like anything? Do they smile at/with the person? ■ Do those providing support talk to the person and ask them questions? ■ Do they have relaxed body language? ■ Do people say hello to the person when they walk into the room? ■ Are staff members sharing the space/room with the person? ■ Do they stand in doorways or sit on the edges of seats rather than be in the same place reciprocating the persons engagement? ■ Do they laugh and joke with the person? ■ Do those providing support talk among themselves without including the person? ■ Does the person know where the people supporting them are, at all times?

Enabling Capable Environments © Pavilion Publishing and Media Ltd and its licensors 2024.

Support for communication	Appraisers should be looking for communication both during structured activities and in more relaxed environments with less structured activities. ■ Do those providing support know the style of communication the person prefers (speech, sign, written, etc.)? ■ Is the person's preferred method of communication being used at all periods throughout the day? ■ Is their preferred communication method to hand (i.e., PECS® board on person, visual communications carried by them or the person supporting them, visual board on walls, objects of reference in a bag that is close by or sitting out for easy access)? ■ Is there regular communication using the persons preferred method? ■ Do those supporting the person understand when the person is communicating a want or need? ■ Are they responsive to the person and their communication style? ■ Do they take the time to understand the persons communication? ■ Are there clear and well-written plans that explain the persons preferred method of communication? ■ Are these plans accessible to everyone who supports them?
Support for participation in meaningful activity	Appraisers should be looking for engagement in all areas of the person's life. This should not simply be at manufactured 'activity times'. ■ Do those supporting the person introduce opportunities for engagement in activities through the person's preferred communication method? ■ Are introductions to new activities staged and tailored to the individual's needs? ■ Do staff use the person's preferred communication during activities to support them to remain engaged? ■ Are they engaged in all areas of their life (leisure, domestic, social, etc)?

Enabling Capable Environments © Pavilion Publishing and Media Ltd and its licensors 2024.

	■ Is the right level of support provided to support engagement? (See Chapter 7) ■ Does the person have regular opportunities to try new activities/tasks? ■ Do others use positive language and an upbeat style when supporting engagement in tasks? ■ Is the person praised for their engagement? ■ Are people encouraged to take the time they need to complete the task? Are they rushed? ■ Are people provided opportunities to take breaks and come back to tasks? Are they made to finish them? Or are tasks completed without the person?
Provision of consistent and predictable environments which honour personalised routines and activities	Appraisers should be looking for consistent practice by others as well as how the person is supported to understand their routines. ■ Are preferred daily and weekly routines detailed in an accessible place for those supporting the person? ■ Are choices for what to do and when respected? ■ Is there flexibility and spontaneity in activities for those who desire this? ■ Are visual/written representations of the person's chosen routines easily accessible to the person? ■ Are people reminded about their routines through their preferred communication method? ■ Are there written documents that provide detailed information on how to complete tasks and activities the way the person prefers? ■ Do others follow these plans? ■ Do others complete tasks/ activities the way they feel works best? ■ Are unavoidable changes discussed with the person and are they offered a favourable alternative?

 Enabling Capable Environments © Pavilion Publishing and Media Ltd and its licensors 2024.

Support to establish and/ or maintain relationships with family and friends	Appraisers should be looking for both physical contact with family, friends, etc. but also other ways the person stays connected to their loved ones such as calls, letters, emails, etc. ■ Do others know who the important people are in the person's life? ■ Do others support the person to arrange seeing/ staying in contact with loved ones regularly (based on the person's preferences)? ■ Do others understand the importance of each relationship to the person? ■ Where appropriate, are contact details and addresses easily accessible to others? ■ Are contact details and addresses accessible to the person? ■ Does the person have access to their preferred communication method with family and friends (i.e., phone, computer, electronic table, letter writing equipment, stamps, etc.)? ■ Do others respect the person's right to have close and intimate relationships with partners while also maintaining the person's safety? ■ Do others support the person to discuss their loved ones? ■ Is the person supported to have access to photographs, memorable items, etc?
Provision of opportunities for choice	Appraisers should be looking for all opportunities the person has to make decisions about their life (from choices about clothing to decisions about how they spend their money). ■ Do staff members understand the types of choices the person would like to make? ■ Are the person's choices respected? ■ Is the person making decisions throughout their day? ■ Does the person have opportunities to make decisions/ choices? ■ Are choices offered to the person using their preferred method of communication?

Enabling Capable Environments © Pavilion Publishing and Media Ltd and its licensors 2024.

	■ Do staff members understand when some choices may overwhelm the person and how to limit this? ■ Is the person involved in making choices in all areas of their life? ■ Do staff members encourage the person to make choices wherever possible? ■ Do they understand how and when the person has made a choice? (This could be through nodding, looking away or towards an item, by walking away, etc.)
Encouragement of more independent functioning	Appraisers should be looking to see if the person is supported to enhance their independence, learn new skills, and try new experiences. ■ Do those providing support understand the importance of choice and control and the impact these have on the person's well-being? ■ Is the person encouraged to learn new skills? ■ Do those providing support try to find opportunities throughout the person's day where they can encourage the person to take more control, try new things, or build their skills? ■ Are there structured written plans for staff members to read that support the person to enhance their independence skills? ■ Are there written goals and outcomes within the person's support plans, Individual Education Plans (IEP), or other paperwork that focus on enhancing their independence? Was the person or their family/friends involved in developing these? ■ Have adaptations been made to the person's environment that supports them to be as independent as possible?
Personal care and health support	Appraisers should be looking to see if the person health and personal care needs are being met. ■ Is the person supported to attend regular medical, dental, and health-related appointments? ■ Do staff members (where appropriate) know the person's medical and health needs? ■ If there are specific health needs, are those supporting the person trained to provide this (i.e., support with conditions such as epilepsy, diabetes, etc.)?

Enabling Capable Environments © Pavilion Publishing and Media Ltd and its licensors 2024.

	■ Is the person able to communicate health or pain needs through their preferred method of communication? ■ Is there easy access to communication aids that support the person's ability to communicate their health needs? ■ Are there detailed plans that staff members can read that would help in understanding if the person was unwell and was unable to communicate this (i.e., DisDAT, support plans, etc.)? ■ Are there processes in place that support the person or staff members to report any health changes or concerns? ■ Are there clearly written plans that detail preferences during personal care routines? Has the person of their family been involved in developing these? ■ Are personal care preferences respected (i.e., specific gender of support worker during routines, certain words used, certain items being present, etc.)?
Provision of an acceptable physical environment	Appraisers should be looking at both the person's home environment but also other environments they may be accessing (i.e., clubs, schools, leisure centres, day centres, etc.)? ■ Do staff members know the person's needs/preferences regarding space, sensory preferences, noise, temperature, lighting, state of repair and safety? ■ Are the person's preferences written and accessible to others who are supporting the person? ■ Are the person's preferences/needs respected? ■ Does the person's home match their preferences/needs? ■ Are they asked about their current physical environment or possible changes to their physical environment? ■ Does the person live where they want and with whom they want? Have they been involved in making that decision?
Mindful, skilled carers	Appraisers should try to identify the knowledge and skills of those supporting the person as well as the opportunities those people have to access training and support. ■ Do those supporting the person know and understand what an intellectual disability is?

Enabling Capable Environments © Pavilion Publishing and Media Ltd and its licensors 2024.

	■ Have they received training in understanding how their intellectual disability may impact on an individual and their needs? ■ Do those supporting the person have the knowledge and skills in implementing person-centred approaches in practice? ■ Is training tailored to the person's specific needs? (Generic communication training is vital as foundational learning but should be enhanced with person-specific training, i.e., PECS, Makaton, etc.). ■ Are those supporting the person provided training in understanding behaviours that challenge and PBS, both generically but also specific to the individual's needs? ■ Is the person and/or their family/friends involved in the development of documents or training in understanding the person and their needs? ■ Are documents reviewed regularly to ensure accuracy? ■ Are there processes in place that allow the identification of new patterns related to behaviours that challenge? Are these followed by swift changes to plans and additional training? ■ Do those who have been trained work in line with the training? Do they ensure they modify the support they provide to prevent behaviours that challenge? ■ Can those who have not been trained easily access training? Has this training been offered, and have they been given the time to access this? ■ Are regular refreshers provided? ■ Do team meetings take place regularly? Do those meetings incorporate learning from PBS training? ■ Is reflective supervision provided regularly?

Enabling Capable Environments © Pavilion Publishing and Media Ltd and its licensors 2024.

Effective management and support	Getting all staff involved will help with this characteristic. It is important that all levels of staff and management are involved in this discussion and that an environment of openness and honesty is created. If the appraiser is in a management role, they may need to consider their own practice and be open to feedback. ■ Do those that manage/oversee those supporting the person have the knowledge and skills to do so? ■ Have they received training in practice leadership, PBS and understanding behaviour, debriefing, reflective practices? ■ Have they been provided with training and support to do this? Do managers receive reflective supervision with their line manager? Do they receive feedback based on observed practice? ■ Do those that manage/oversee those supporting the person understand capable environments, know how to support its development, and how to monitor progress? ■ Are those supporting the person led well? ■ Do managers hold high values regarding the rights of people with intellectual disabilities and do they focus on quality of life? Do they work in a way that promotes this? ■ Do managers 'walk the talk' and are they observed acting in ways they promote to staff teams (i.e., respecting choices of supported people, following plans, responding to behaviours that challenge in a respectful manner and in line with any plans, reflecting and changing practice based on this)? ■ Are those supporting the person able to easily get access to advice, guidance and support from their manager? ■ Are those supporting the person given regular feedback about their practice? Are they coached and mentored in new areas or areas of development? ■ Are those supporting the person supervised regularly? Does their supervision involve discussions about quality of life (see Chapter 1), practice, new support plans, understanding behaviours that challenge, PBS?

Enabling Capable Environments © Pavilion Publishing and Media Ltd and its licensors 2024.

Effective organisational context	Appraisers will need to review their organisational context. They may choose to work with their manager to complete this section. ■ Are the organisation's policies and procedures informed by a focus of the rights of people with an intellectual disability, person-centred values, and PBS? ■ Are organisational outcomes linked to people's well-being and quality of life? ■ Is the reduction of restrictive practices a key aim of the organisation? ■ Does the organisation recognise the communicative intent of behaviours that challenge? ■ Does the organisation encourage and offer training in human rights, a person-centred approach, and PBS?

Thinking space

Before beginning your meetings, observations and review of practice, you should take time to consider:

1. What is the best way to make sure you get a full picture of all the people supporting the person? This is usually best done by spending time in practice.
2. How much time will you allocate to conduct meetings and observations?
3. Will you ask others to help? (If so, how will you ensure they are skilled in the Capable Environments Appraisal?)
4. What times of the day will you ensure you capture? (How will you ensure you gain a good understanding of the person's daily support?)
5. Which paperwork or documents will you review? How much time will this take?

The 'Capable Environments Appraisal' is provided as an appendix at the end of this book. This can be copied to facilitate the appraisal process.

Enabling Capable Environments © Pavilion Publishing and Media Ltd and its licensors 2024.

Case study

In Hume *et al.* (2021), after completing the appraisal, the authors supported frontline managers to review the findings and use this to create specific capable environment plans for each supported person. Each supported person had a plan which detailed the ten characteristics of a capable environment which should be implemented for that person every day. Characteristics 11 and 12 were not included in this stage of plan development as they were not specific to the individual, but a focus was placed on these through other training and advocacy projects such as working closely with senior management to make changes to policies and drive towards increasing knowledge and skills through training. An example of one plan within one section of the table is shown below.

Table 2.3: Capable environments plan example

Support for participation in meaningful activity	To support Sam to engage in an activity, staff should follow the guidelines below. ■ Staff should direct Sam to his symbol strip with the activity he is about to engage in. ■ Staff should prompt him by saying 'Sam, time for…', while showing him the symbol. ■ Staff should use a positive tone of voice and open body language. ■ Staff should give Sam time to process what has been said and decide whether he wants to do this. ■ Staff should go with Sam to where the activity is. ■ Staff should also engage in the activity alongside Sam. Sam enjoys activities when others engage with him and are enjoying themselves. ■ If Sam is distracted, prompt him back on task (say 'Sam, [the activity] first, then [the next task]) * If Sam is indicating he wants to stop the activity, respect that decision. ■ Staff should use graduated guidance (see Chapter 7) to support Sam to achieve the task without taking over.

Enabling Capable Environments © Pavilion Publishing and Media Ltd and its licensors 2024.

	■ Staff should praise Sam throughout the activity. Be specific about what you are praising ('Sam, well done playing the drums, that sounds lovely', or, 'Sam well done waiting in the queue', etc.). ■ When the task is complete, staff should tell Sam the activity is finished and should direct him to his symbol strip to indicate what is next ('Sam, [the activity] is finished, time for [next activity]) ■ Again, praise Sam for his participation. Sam loves high fives and fist bumps. ■ Sam likes to send pictures of what he has been doing to his family and friends. Ask Sam to take a picture on his phone and remind him that we can send these later. After any activity, it is important for you to assess if there is a need for Sam to have some chill-out time or if he requires a 'filler' activity. You should have several smaller activities that you can engage in with Sam, such as having a cup of coffee, listening to music, reading magazines, etc. This will ensure that Sam receives lots of your time and attention throughout the day.

Reviewing the appraisal and developing opportunities into plans

After completing the appraisal, there will likely be a few achievements that are already occurring in the person's support. It is important to highlight the great work that is already occurring.

There will likely also be several opportunities to enhance the person's support and enable the environment to be more capable. This can feel daunting at first, especially if you attempt to achieve all of these at once. Start small, move slow (LaVigna, 1994). It is important to agree on what the priorities are and begin from there; the idea is to practice this and get used to this way of working. Therefore, it's fine to start with a couple of opportunities initially. This will grow as you progress, ensuring all characteristics of the capable environment are being met.

Enabling Capable Environments © Pavilion Publishing and Media Ltd and its licensors 2024.

Thinking space

Consider how you will decide which opportunities to work on initially and which can be addressed later?

- Are there any opportunities that you know will bring immediate fun to the person's life? This should be first.
- Are there any pressing matters?
- Do those that support the person have a desire to focus on a specific area?
- Are there areas that can be addressed quickly?

Who will help you make that decision?

- Can the person choose which opportunities are priorities?
- Can their family/friends?
- Can those that support the person be involved?

Discussing the opportunities with the full staff team

After deciding which opportunities will be the focus, you will then need to decide how you will communicate these opportunities to the staff team.

Some opportunities may already be plans within the person's support plan or Individual Education Plan. These may need to be reviewed to ensure enough detail has been provided. Others may be new, and you may need to work collaboratively to develop a written and detailed support plan for that opportunity. Others may be things such as ensuring a percentage of staff are trained in the person's communication preferences or Positive Behaviour Support (PBS); this may need to be recorded in staff development records and reviewed regularly.

Enabling Capable Environments © Pavilion Publishing and Media Ltd and its licensors 2024.

Methods to support the enablement of capable environments

Case study

In Hume *et al*. (2021), the authors developed and implemented a Periodic Service Review (PSR) to support the implementation of the ten capable environment characteristics (see Chapter 5 for more information). Each characteristic was developed into a PSR standard, which stated:

- What the desired performance is.
- When it is expected to occur.
- Who is responsible for ensuring it happens.
- How we will know it has been done.

Below is an example of a PSR standard.

Table 2.4: Capable environments PSR standard example

Standard
What is the desired performance? (What is it that we want to see happen. Keep this simple. For example, two observations to be completed.) *Staff are observed using Sam's now-and-next communication strip when supporting him to move between tasks/activities.*
When is it expected to occur? (This is how often you want to see the performance happen. For example, daily, every week.) *An observation should take place at least once a day.*
Who is responsible? (Who will be required to ensure this happens. For example, frontline manager, shift lead?) *The person leading the shift to conduct an observation every day.*
How will it be verified? (There are two ways this can be done.1: Permanent product. This is a physical thing that shows something has been completed. 2: Direct observation.) *Seven observation sheets to be reviewed each week. Observations should detail the use/non-use of the now and next communication strip. Frontline manager to review observation sheets each week.*

 Enabling Capable Environments © Pavilion Publishing and Media Ltd and its licensors 2024.

It is important to note that the observation forms should be reviewed regularly but if you had identified early in the process that this was not occurring, you would address this at this stage and not wait until the scheduled time had concluded. This is a dynamic process, and the focus is always moving forward to achieving the standard.

In their programme (Hume *et al* 2021), all ten standards were placed in one document as a guide for those who support the person and those who manage/ oversee them. At the front of the document was a Capable Environments PSR sheet (see Appendix Two: Capable Environments Periodic Service Review Sheet). This sheet was used daily by the manager to identify whether the ten characteristics were being met. The manager would observe a standard being met or review physical documents that indicated whether a standard had been met. The 'Capable Environments PSR sheet' was completed by marking an '😊' for the standard being achieved or an 'O' for an opportunity for the future. An average of these was calculated each week and added to a graph. This was displayed visually in staff rooms to support staff in understanding how many capable environment characteristics were being achieved and whether this was progressing on a week-by-week basis.

Monitoring the opportunities

Using a PSR is a great way to bring the ten characteristics together in one place. This will help those who support the person to know which ten opportunities are being prioritised.

Each of the ten outcomes you have created also needs to be appraised to ensure progress is being made and staff are provided with the support and feedback to achieve them. A PSR is a great tool for facilitating this.

Enabling Capable Environments © Pavilion Publishing and Media Ltd and its licensors 2024.

Thinking space

Take some time to think about why ongoing support and review is required for enhancing the characteristics of a capable environment.

Think about a time a new process or plan was implemented in your school or workplace.

- How did you know what the plans were?
- How did you know if you were following the plan correctly?
- How did you know if the plan was working well?

Support plans can be difficult to understand and implement. That is why those implementing the plans need training, support, coaching and feedback. We all need to know if what we are doing is correct and if it is having the impact we want it to have.

Opportunities: coaching and mentoring

When you begin implementing the PSR, those who support the person will need help and guidance to enhance their skills to meet the capable environment characteristic. You are likely to have many 'Os' – opportunities to enhance characteristics. Coaching and mentoring are vital to developing a capable environment (see Chapter 6).

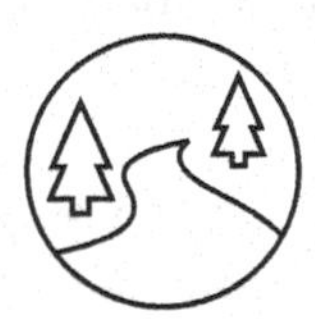

Paving the way to success

Implementing and maintaining capable environments will take time. There may be occasions when you are faced with challenges to implementing new plans, a feeling that there is a lack of progress or a return to old ways of working. Below are some ways to support yourself throughout the process.

Time – plan enough time between each stage:

- This will allow for breathing and thinking space when things may not go to plan.
- This will allow for time for others to ask questions and for you to be able to work in a collaborative way to address these questions.

 Enabling Capable Environments © Pavilion Publishing and Media Ltd and its licensors 2024.

Hurdles – don't be disheartened:

- There may be times when great plans do not work well or staff teams are struggling to try new things. This is part of the process. Take your time to work through these together.
- There may be bumps in the road and periods where PSR scores are lower than previous times. The PSR will help you to identify what is not working and will support collaborative teamwork to enhance this in the future.

Seek help and support:

- Don't do it all on your own. Remember to link closely with those who can drive and implement changes and provide support to overcome difficulties together in your specific work or home environment.
- Capable environments should never sit with one individual; it is important to work collaboratively and support all parties to take ownership of the process.

Discussion questions

Below are some possible questions you are likely to be asked or you will ask during the process of creating capable environments.

1. We have tried these things before, and they didn't work. Why will it work this time?

   Remind everyone that at the heart of what you are doing is the person. Stress that everyone coming together and working collaboratively for the same goal will make a difference in capable environments being taken forward. Emphasise that each characteristic of capable environments has thorough evidence and research to show its impact on quality of life and behaviour that challenges.

2. I'm already very busy, will this give me more work to do?

   There may be some initial work to set up the systems and processes, but in the long run, the person's quality of life will increase. Capable environments have been found to enhance the work environment for staff and managers.

3. I don't want to be watched doing my job. Will I be judged?

   Explore the importance of observations in enhancing skills and addressing difficulties. Remind everyone that there will be a focus on both the things that are being done well and that should continue, as well as some of the opportunities that can be increased. Make sure to discuss all the positives that have been found after the appraisal has taken place.

4. What is a capable environment?

   ✔ It is a framework that focuses on increasing the quality of support and therefore the quality of life of those being supported.

   ✔ It is completed in partnership with everyone involved in a person's life.

   ✘ It is not an auditing tool/process.

   ✘ It is not implemented to criticise or catch people out.

Conclusion

- Capable environments help move the focus to what we all need to do, to better meet and coordinate a person's needs; it begins with a focus towards changing the 'challenging environments' around the person.
- The capable environments approach 'promises substantial quality of life improvements for individuals, better work environments for staff and a reduction in the costs associated with specialist care and out-of-area placements' (McGill *et al.*, 2020).
- Challenging behaviour is more likely to occur in environments that are disorganised, that fail to promote quality of life outcomes and that are unresponsive to personal needs; therefore, addressing such 'environmental deficits' by ensuring environments are more capable would be a rational foundation for support design irrespective of the presence of behaviour that challenges and, more importantly, ensuring our attention is focused on ecological manipulations that smooth the fit between the person and their environment (Carr *et al.*, 1996 & LaVigna *et al.*, 2022).
- Studies show that 'many of the environments where individuals at risk of displaying challenging behaviour are supported are not nearly as capable as they could be' (McGill *et al.*, 2022).
- Capable environments are a collection of 12 characteristics. Each characteristic, when implemented, is associated with improvements to quality of life, quality of support and a reduction in the occurrence of challenging behaviour. Each

Enabling Capable Environments © Pavilion Publishing and Media Ltd and its licensors 2024.

characteristic comes with an established evidence base of what matters in quality of support and quality of life (McGill *et al.*, 2022).

- Before enabling an environment to become more capable, it is important to understand the capability of the environment currently. Using the capable environment characteristics is an effective way of appraising the current environment to identify achievements being made and opportunities for development (Hume *et al.*, 2021).
- After completing the appraisal, there will likely be several opportunities to enhance the person's support and make their environment more capable. Using a Periodic Service Review (PSR) is a great way to prioritise where to start collaboratively and to monitor progress in enabling a capable environment (Hume *et al.*, 2021).

Enabling Capable Environments © Pavilion Publishing and Media Ltd and its licensors 2024.

Chapter 3: Applying capable environments: optimising individual and personalised supports

'The social and physical environment provided by services constitutes the main means by which services can improve the behaviour and lifestyle of service users. The task is no less than the design of a culture which will support clients in living quality lifestyles.' (Emerson *et al*., 1994)

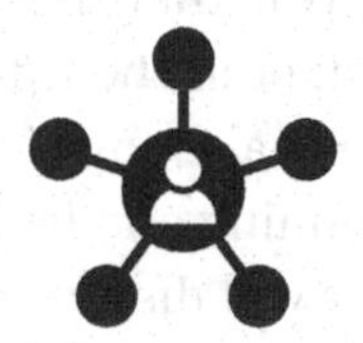

Chapter contents:

- Positive social interaction.
- Support for communication.
- Support for participation in meaningful activity.
- Provision of consistent and predictable environments which honour personalised routines and activities.
- Support to establish and maintain relationships with family and friends.
- Provision of opportunities for choice.
- Encouragement of more independent functioning.
- Personal care and health support.

Learning outcomes

After reading this chapter and completing the suggested activities and reflection, the reader should be able to:

- Recognise the features of eight components of a capable environment.
- Understand how these components are applied in practice.
- Collaborate with others to optimise people's support, enabling them to be more capable.
- Review current practices and identify opportunities to optimise personalised supports.

Introduction

In Chapter 2 we discussed the 12 characteristics of capable environments. We established that when implemented well, this will create an enabling and capable environment, an environment that increases quality of life, which in turn can contribute to a reduction in behaviours that challenge. Eight of these characteristics are indicators of support that those working directly with the person can influence, change and adapt in their daily practice. The remaining four are supports that require more of a change in the system (organisation) and therefore may take a little more planning and longer to influence if they are applied in practice (Chapter 4). This chapter will discuss in more depth how eight of the capable environment's characteristics that apply to direct support staff can enhance their everyday practice. We will share examples from our experience and will provide practical examples of how the characteristics of capable environments can be embedded into practice in your home, educational setting or support service.

Positive social interaction

Positive Social Interaction

We speak at length during this book about the need for people with an intellectual disability to be actively engaged and to be advocates in their own lives. How successfully this is facilitated for an individual is dependent on many factors. One of the most important of those is social interaction. This is outlined as:

> *'In situations where the person receives unconditional, positive social interactions they are less likely to display challenging behaviour to obtain*

Enabling Capable Environments © Pavilion Publishing and Media Ltd and its licensors 2024.

> *social interaction; carers who establish good relationships with individuals can embed any necessary less positive interactions (e.g. physical care that may be uncomfortable or distressing). Most people (with and without learning disabilities) want to receive positive social interactions from those around them.'* (McGill *et al*, 2020 p4)

As individuals, we are inherently social, and most people want to have positive social interactions with those around them. This can make the difference between someone having a good day or a bad day. We are all aware of how it feels when someone interacts with us in a warm, positive manner and in a way that we are comfortable with. Conversely, we also know how it feels when someone interacts with us in a cold or rude manner. These types of interactions have a huge effect on how we feel about ourselves and what we may or may not want to do with that person in the future.

We know that people with an intellectual disability:

- Encounter disproportionate levels of loneliness.
- Experience a lack of meaningful social connections.
- Have a smaller social circle of people with whom they can interact.

It is often the case that interactions within settings where people require support are task-driven. For example, contact or connection with the person being supported is often limited to times when others need to give instruction or prompts for set tasks, i.e. 'It's time for dinner', 'We need to go shopping'. While this may be important in supporting someone to understand what is happening or what could be done next, it is the quality of these interactions that is crucial to making a positive interaction that is more likely to be reciprocated. Only experiencing the types of social interactions that are task- or instruction-driven can negatively impact relationships and well-being.

Thinking space

Consider the following: a staff member is going to find out what someone that they are supporting would like for breakfast.

Scenario 1: They knock on the person's door and wait to be invited in. Once invited in they say, 'Good morning, how are you feeling today?' and wait for the person to respond. They then ask, 'What would you like for breakfast today?' Once the person replies, they say, 'Great, when you're ready we can go to the kitchen and make it together'.

Consider the same scenario with a different interactional style.

Scenario 2: The staff member enters the person's room without knocking and says, 'Your breakfast's on the table' and leaves.

- Which interactional style would you prefer to be part of?
- How would scenario 1 make you feel in comparison to scenario 2?
- Would you be encouraged or enthused to want to get up and engage in scenario 2?

Why are positive interactions important?

How we interact with people is one of the factors that sets the scene for interactions and establishing rapport that can impact someone's quality of life both positively and negatively. Spending time with someone in a natural way without the requirement for a person to always be expected to do something is vital. Sitting and listening to music together, having a conversation about a shared interest, checking to see if they are okay, and actively listening when they are talking can all have a hugely positive impact. By contrast: leaving people alone for long periods, ignoring someone when they attempt to communicate, and only interacting to provide instructions or ask for things to be done hurts a person's self-esteem and sense of feeling being valued. When people's attempts to socially interact or connect with others are frequently ignored and rejected this deprives the person of basic social connections and can lead to social isolation and poor physical and emotional well-being (Beadle-Brown *et al.*, 2014, 2015).

Enabling Capable Environments © Pavilion Publishing and Media Ltd and its licensors 2024.

Thinking space

In our clinical practice, we sometimes hear teams saying, 'Oh, we're busy! We can't respond every time someone is trying to get our attention.'

Perhaps people are very busy and cannot respond in a way the person needs immediately, but how would you respond to a friend who waved at you at a train station seeking your attention when you were 'busy' rushing to catch your train? Would you ignore them? Tell them to go and do something else? Say you are too busy for them?

Or would you:

- Wave back smiling and saying, 'Lovely to see you will call you later – got to run for my train!'?
- Decide you can catch the next train and go have coffee with your friend?
- Send them a text 'Sorry I missed you, catch you next time' with lots of emoji hearts?

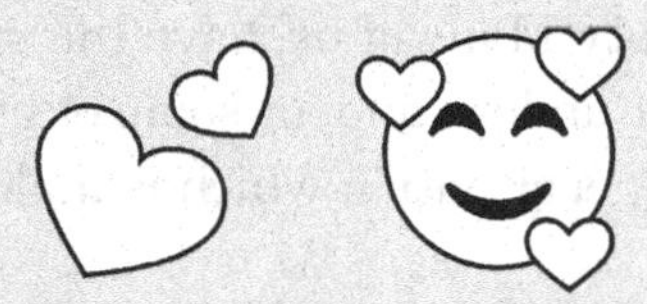

In this situation you are maintaining a positive relationship with someone you have respect for.

Use this thinking space to reflect on our daily interactions with people.

Do you think people feel valued and respected?

Positive social interactions can lead people to engage more, leading to better outcomes in terms of skill development and emotional well-being. Emotional well-being is connected to feeling contented, a lack of stress and having a positive self-identity, and one way that we can influence how people feel about themselves is through our interactions with them. When we consider interaction through this lens, it shows just how important it is for us to always be mindful of how we engage with people not only through what we say but also through how we behave (Bigby & Bould 2017).

Support for communication

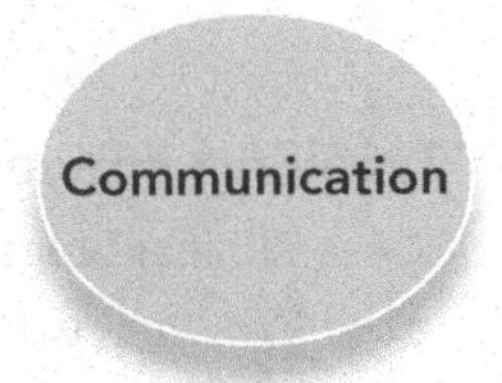

McGill *et al.* (2020) explains that 'support for communication' is important as:

> *'Challenging behaviour is less likely when the person understands and is understood by those around them. Most people (with and without learning disabilities) want to communicate with those around them, especially those they are close to.'* (p4)

Being able to communicate your wants and needs is essential for everyone. If we think back to the reasons that behaviours that challenge may occur, we should consider it is likely to be that there is an unmet need being communicated (although not always intentional communication). We are sure we can all think of occasions where we have been unable to fully explain ourselves and have become frustrated. Being able to understand what is expected of us in any given situation is also important. Imagine being placed in a new environment with expectations you don't know or understand and that haven't been explained to you. This would likely cause a lot of stress and anxiety. Many of us, have the means of communication to say we are confused and don't understand, or some of us may take the opportunity to make our excuses and leave a situation which is making us anxious.

In our experience, many people with an intellectual disability (but not all) will have some communication support needs and may have worked closely with a speech and language therapist. There may be well-written documents that detail the person's preferred communication methods. Unfortunately, this does not always transfer to these communication supports being used correctly or consistently (Johnson *et al.*, 2012). It's important to consider why this occurs:

- At times, others can believe the person being supported no longer needs communication support or aid. When considering whether a person no longer needs a communication system, it is important to remind those supporting them not to abandon any current methods until a qualified professional can assess and provide access to a new communication system. Providing nothing at all or a communication system that doesn't work for the person could lead to confusion and distress.
- Some may feel the person now knows their routines and the communication supports and aids are not required. When addressing those who suggest that communication supports are not required due to the person knowing their routines, it is important to remind them that the person may be struggling to

 Enabling Capable Environments © Pavilion Publishing and Media Ltd and its licensors 2024.

remember their routines without this support. In addition, if the communication system is abandoned, how can we support the person to access new spaces, create new routines and expand their experiences if they choose to?

- Those supporting the person may not have received training in using the person's preferred method of communication. A lack of knowledge and experience in using the person's communication method could result in the method being abandoned. Regular training focused on the person's preferred communication method should be delivered to those who support the person. Any new person who is introduced to the person and will be expected to communicate with them regularly should also receive this training and have time to shadow those who use the method well.
- Written support plans or assessments may be technical and difficult to follow. Written documentation must be provided in a way that all those supporting the person will understand. It is beneficial to avoid jargon and focus on language that describes what the person should do.
- Some communication supports require regular maintenance such as printing and laminating, updating software on electronic tablets, or the need to purchase new physical items due to wear and tear, making these supports difficult to maintain. Maintaining communication systems can cause some difficulties. There must be several people who know how and when to update any communication aids. These people should be given the time and resources to do this.

The above factors must be considered and revisited regularly to ensure the person always has the right communication support and aids.

Support for participation in meaningful activity

Engagement in Meaningful Activity

McGill *et al.* (2020) state that:

> *'Challenging behaviour is less likely when the person is meaningfully occupied. Skilled support ensures that they can participate at least partially even in relatively complex activities so that they learn to cope with demands and difficulties that might otherwise provoke challenging behaviour. Most people (with and without learning disabilities) like to be busy.'* (p5)

Enabling Capable Environments © Pavilion Publishing and Media Ltd and its licensors 2024.

Engaging in meaningful activity is important for us all. Imagine a life where all or most activities are done for you, and you are a passive recipient. Yes, that does seem appealing initially, when you think about your busy life and the limited free time you may have but imagine you didn't have a busy life. Imagine that every task in your whole life was done for you. What would you be doing? Would this become monotonous?

Engaging in meaningful activities provides opportunities to engage with others, learn new skills, gain pride in what you can do, and increase self-esteem. For many of us, our busy lives are filled with activities and people we like.

Meaningful activity can include:

- Being actively involved in creating and maintaining a homely environment.
- Accessing leisure activities.
- Engaging in hobbies.
- Having people to talk to and share activities with.
- Going to places where you feel welcomed and included.
- Learning new skills.

Enhancing opportunities for people to be actively involved in their lives begins with knowing what is important to them and then using this information to shape and plan with people what their day will look like to ensure any opportunities are not missed or overlooked. This should keep us focused on what is important to the person rather than what we think is important.

Enabling Capable Environments © Pavilion Publishing and Media Ltd and its licensors 2024.

Thinking space

Think about a colleague or friend who has different interests from you. Maybe they love to cycle, crochet or bake, and what is meaningful to them is engaging in this task multiple times a week. What if they were supporting you and decided this should be a meaningful activity for you and expected you to do this multiple times a week? How would you feel? Would this suddenly become meaningful to you?

Now imagine you enjoyed an activity such as painting, gardening or pottery and gained a lot from engaging in this activity. What if someone that had no interest in this task or who didn't consider it beneficial decided that this should not be part of your life? How would you feel?

When we support individuals with intellectual disabilities, we also need to consider the tasks or activities in their lives that may not appear to be meaningful to others but that have a huge impact on their lives and well-being. For some people, engaging in repetitive actions or activities that provide sensory feedback is meaningful and should be respected. We should never place our preconceptions on other people.

You must put aside your perceptions of what 'meaningful' means and come together with the person to find out what they find meaningful. So how can you do this?

Ask the person what is important to them, what they like, enjoy or want to try. This can seem very simple but, for many people, just asking, particularly using only verbal language, will not help them to consider what is important to them and if they would like more of this in their lives. There are some things you can do rather than using a verbal request:

1. Use the person's preferred communication method when asking these questions (pictures, PECS, sign, written information, Talking Mats, etc.).
2. Limit the number of questions being posed at one time and do not overcomplicate what you are asking.
3. Do not expect to get all the answers in one conversation. This may take time and may change based on new information. Seeking what is meaningful to a person should be part of what we do every day when we are supporting someone with an intellectual disability, not only one conversation at a set time.

4. If the person has never accessed some experiences, they may be unable to tell you if this is important to them. You will need to consider how you can introduce them to these experiences at a pace and in a way that works for them (i.e. talking about your experience of the activity, sharing others' experiences of an activity, videos, pictures, drop-in sessions where the person can dip in and out as they choose).
5. Be observant and watch the person's body language and how they respond and interact with experiences. Check-in with the person after these experiences.
6. How does the person spend their time? Do they appear engaged and happy?
7. Speak to those who know the person well. What have they found is meaningful to the person? Check this with the person to make sure and confirm.

Once you know what is important and meaningful to the person it is important to ensure people supporting the individual know how to plan for these activities to increase access and engagement in a way that is positive and meaningful to them. Chapter 7 provides detailed guidance on how to support engagement and participation, increase choice and offer opportunities to try new experiences.

Provision of consistent and predictable environments which honour personalised routines and activities

Consistent and Predictable Environments

'...challenging behaviour is more likely when the person is supported inconsistently or when in transition between one activity/environment and another activity/environment. Most people (with and without learning disabilities) value consistent and predictable support.' (McGill *et al*., 2020, p5)

Understanding what is going to happen and when is important to us all. Imagine working in an environment where the rules or routines change every day, those you work with vary regularly, your manager's expectations of what you should be doing and when alter, and you aren't told about this in advance. This would be an extremely stressful environment. Now think about how this might feel for people with intellectual disabilities whose routines are changed with no explanation, the routines that have been created have been developed for others' benefits and preferences rather than their own, and possibly those supporting them are not

Enabling Capable Environments © Pavilion Publishing and Media Ltd and its licensors 2024.

well known to them and don't use their preferred communication methods. We also want you to imagine this happening not just during an eight-hour working day but during your full day, within your own home.

At times and for many reasons we can get into habits of working in ways that better meet the needs of ourselves, managers and the service rather than those we support. Working in this way does not provide person-centred support. It is important to understand each person's individual preferences in their routines and activities. This can be achieved through:

- Asking the person using verbal language.
- Using Talking Mats™ or other alternative communication systems to gain the person's opinions.
- Observing the person during their activities and routines. Watching for responses that may indicate they enjoy it (smiling, relaxed body language, etc.) or that they do not (tense, look upset, etc).
- Reviewing records and speaking to people who spent time with the person to identify if there are set times of the day or particular activities in which the individual is actively engaged or becomes distressed.

  ('Five good communication standards', Royal College of Speech and Language Therapists, 2016.)

From this information daily, weekly and/or monthly planners should be developed that meet those preferences. These should be developed in line with the person's preferred communication method and should be displayed or provided to the person in a way that works for them. Some examples of this are:

- A calendar on the wall with pictures or written words that detail what is happening, when it is happening and with whom.
- A daily, weekly or monthly written diary (with written language or pictures).
- A visual board on the wall with pictures indicating what is scheduled for the day, week or month.
- 'Now and next' or 'now, next and later' boards. These are visual, hand-held aids that detail what two or three immediate tasks are planned or will be taking place.
- Digital versions of all the above on hand-held electronic devices.

Enabling Capable Environments © Pavilion Publishing and Media Ltd and its licensors 2024.

Along with these communication supports, written support plans or guidelines that detail how the person likes to be supported during each activity should be developed and easily accessible to everyone who supports them during these tasks. These written guidelines should detail:

- The specific steps that should be followed within each activity or task.
- The types and level of support that the person would like during that activity.
- The communication methods that should be used.
- How to promote choice.
- The ways the person may indicate they want things to happen later, change or stop.

Those working with the person should be encouraged to review these written guidelines regularly. Even after these plans are in place it is important to continuously go back to the person and check that the plans are working for them. Remember, preferences change, and we should adapt our support to meet the person's needs and wishes. It is essential to ensure that those who support the person understand when and how the person makes choices and that those supporting the person respect the choices and make changes based on this. Remember, changing our minds is okay and it's important that the people we support also have this right.

After a time, teams may feel that they are very familiar with how to provide support and may not refer to support plans or guidelines. This can risk parts of the plan being missed or skipped. An example of this might be people stopping using the picture for the gym and just verbally suggesting it – if the person needs a visual prompt to understand what is happening then a key part of the support plan is missed.

Regularly checking that plans are being implemented as stated is key to ensuring consistency and predictability. This can be achieved through:

- Observations of activities (where you ask someone to watch what is going on and give you feedback).
- Reviewing support plans and the person's participation (do the plans still work, are you getting feedback from the person that they still enjoy what they are doing?)

 Enabling Capable Environments © Pavilion Publishing and Media Ltd and its licensors 2024.

- Regularly discussing the support plans and guidelines at person-centred planning meetings and reviews, at team meetings and supervision, making changes where required while reviewing this with the person being supported.

Thinking space

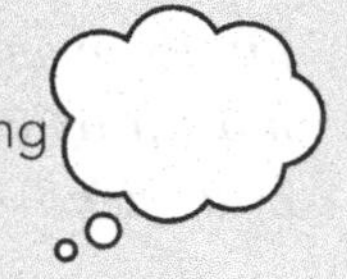

Consider a routine you engage in most days. This could be your morning routine, your weekly visit to see a friend or family member or a weekly karate class.

Think about the different steps involved in the activity itself or the steps involved in getting ready for the activity (the order you like to do things, packing bags with essential items, preparing a dish, planning a route or travel, etc.). Now imagine someone decides you should do this in a different order because they know it will be best for you or because it is easier for them.

Would you be happy to change your routines for their routines?

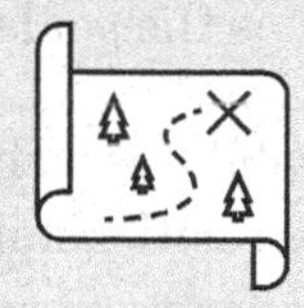

Having a plan for a personalised routine is a little like having a road map. Think about an activity you do that is important to you. If you needed someone to make sure this activity happened in a certain way, what are the steps they would need to follow?

When writing your plan, you may want to think about some of the following:

- When it needs to happen?
- What you need to get you to the activity
- Are there any resources you need, money, certain clothing etc.?
- Do you need assistance to participate in the activity?

Then reflect on the plans or guidelines in your service, do they provide enough detail and steps to guide people on what to do to ensure routines are personalised and written in a way to ensure success?

The people we support must decide how they want to live their lives. It is our role to ensure we understand what that means for them and provide this consistently.

Support to establish and maintain relationships with family and friends

Relationships with Family and Friends

'...challenging behaviour is less likely when the person is with family members or others with whom they have positive relationships. For most people (with and without learning disabilities), relationships with family and friends are a central part of their life.' (McGill *et al*, 2020, p5)

Try to think of a time when you didn't have your family and closest friends around you for an extended period. Maybe you had moved to a new country or were away from home for the first time and didn't yet have strong relationships with those around you. You might feel lost, lonely and possibly scared. Our close friends and/or family are important to us all. If lucky, these relationships are fundamental and provide us with love and safety. In addition, these relationships are usually long-lasting and are with people who know our history, the challenges we have faced, the achievements we have made, as well as the goals we seek for the future.

For many people with intellectual disabilities who are supported by those who are not immediate friends or family, these relationships are even more crucial. For many, the people who support them may change regularly (as they move on to new roles or jobs), the people who support them may not have been chosen by them and may be people they would not choose to spend time with. Often staff who are in paid roles are told there is a need to maintain professional boundaries meaning our relationships with people are different; we don't share parts of our lives as we would do with our friends and family. This means that relationships with family and friends should be prioritised for people with an intellectual disability and, where required, people should be supported to maintain these. To do this we need to know:

- Who is important to the person?
- How can the person or others access these people?
- What communication methods do they like to use to stay in contact?
- How often they would both like to see and/or contact one another?

Imagine you are in a new country with no friends or family, what might you do? Some people might:

- Phone or video call family and friends.
- Write letters or emails.

Enabling Capable Environments © Pavilion Publishing and Media Ltd and its licensors 2024.

- Look through physical or electronic photo albums.
- Make new friends to share some time with.
- Plan a visit to see friends or family.
- Invite people to their house for dinner.
- Go away for a weekend break with them.

Facilitating contact with family and friends is crucial to the well-being of people with an intellectual disability. There are many ways to do this, as highlighted above. If you are supporting someone who does not live with family or close friends, it is important to recognise how important these relationships are and ensure this is prioritised.

Love, sex and intimate relationships are also important for people with intellectual disabilities. Most people in a relationship see their partner regularly and choose how and when this happens. However, for people with an intellectual disability, this is more difficult as they may be reliant on others to access a way to visit a partner. They may not have enough support hours to visit and spend time with a loved one whenever they want to. The organisation's policies and training may be only focused on being risk averse, for example, a narrative that people with an intellectual disability cannot consent to intimate relationships or that they don't need them!

Organisations must adhere to legislation based on safeguarding where the issue of consent is discussed in detail. However, this needs to be balanced with the person's needs, wishes and right to have relationships. There are some very helpful resources available at www.supportedloving.org.uk.

Provision of opportunities for choice

Opportunities for Choice

> *'...challenging behaviour is less likely when the person is doing things that they have chosen to do or with people that they have chosen to be with. Most people (with and without learning disabilities) value the opportunity to decide things for themselves.'* (McGill *et al.*, 2020, p6)

To understand the impact of making choices, we need to understand its importance to someone's quality of life. We all make lots of choices in our lives. The choices we make can determine the quality and direction of our day and our life. Some

Enabling Capable Environments © Pavilion Publishing and Media Ltd and its licensors 2024.

people with an intellectual disability do not get the opportunity to make choices. The reality for a lot of people with an intellectual disability is that choices which directly impact their lives are often made without their involvement, instead of with them or by them. This may be significant life choices such as where they live, how their finances are managed, who supports them, as well as everyday choices such as what clothing they will wear, what they will eat and what type of activities they will do.

Thinking space

Consider the following scenarios:

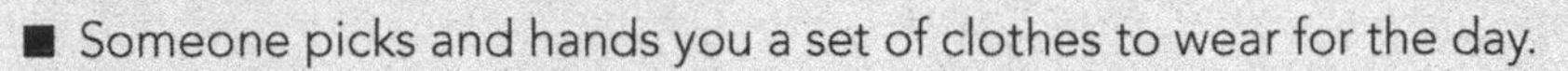

- Someone picks and hands you a set of clothes to wear for the day.

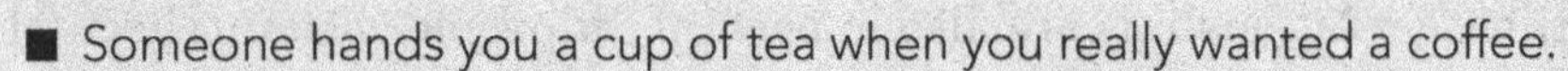

- Someone hands you a cup of tea when you really wanted a coffee.

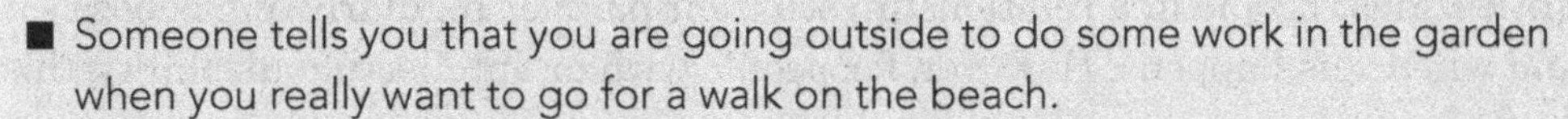

- Someone tells you that you are going outside to do some work in the garden when you really want to go for a walk on the beach.

Now consider the lack of control you have in these scenarios and discuss the following:

- How would this make you feel?
- How willing would you be to continue to engage in these interactions?
- What impact would this have on the overall quality of your life?

When people are afforded choice and control over things that impact their own lives, it can lead to higher levels of engagement. This is particularly important for people with an intellectual disability who spend a disproportionate amount of time disengaged. We need to remember that people with an intellectual disability have the right to choose, it is not something that should be earned or given **it is a right**, and our support should be framed as respecting this right and acting in a way that enables this right to choose.

People have the right to have power and control over their own lives. It ensures greater opportunities for people to be involved in things that matter to them and reduces the frustration associated with having others make decisions for them. Making choices ensures people are not treated as being passive and dependent, rather they are in control. This is discussed in more detail in Chapter 7.

For choices to be meaningful in someone's life, they have to be significant to them. We must take the time to find out what people are interested in and motivated by.

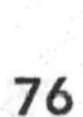

Enabling Capable Environments © Pavilion Publishing and Media Ltd and its licensors 2024.

This allows for choice to be real, functional and in context with the person's life. When thinking about how to promote choices to someone it is important to understand how the person communicates and their level of understanding. For example, asking open questions such as 'What do you want to do today?' may be too overwhelming or abstract for some people. It is important to provide the correct structure for the person to understand the choices and make informed decisions. This may be about the number of choices offered (a choice between two options, for example), or how the choice is presented (verbally, written, using pictures, signs, symbols or objects). Taking the time to find out how someone processes information and knowing how to introduce that information in a meaningful way can make the difference between someone actively engaging in making choices for themselves and not.

Encouragement of more independent functioning

Independent Functioning

> *McGill et al. (2020) stress that support to increase independent functioning is vital: '...the development of new skills and independent functioning enables the individual to have more control over their life. Most people (with and without learning disabilities) like to be independent'* (p6).

Think about a skill you have learned. What impact did this have on your life? How did learning this new skill increase your independence? How did doing this make you feel?

From a young age, we strive to learn new things and be independent. How many times have you tried to help a toddler with something only to be met with a clear, 'I can do it myself' response? We are driven to learn how to do things and do them well with a sense of pride and purpose. We discussed earlier in this chapter the need for personalised routines and choices. One of the most effective ways to make these a reality is to ensure people have the opportunity to learn how to do things for themselves when and where they choose to.

So, being independent is a core factor in having control over our lives. However, we need to consider when and how people are supported to learn and use new skills in a way that is right for them. This is discussed in more detail in Chapter 8, but for now, we will consider some examples of how learning a new skill can increase independence:

Enabling Capable Environments © Pavilion Publishing and Media Ltd and its licensors 2024.

- Imagine being a young child and learning how to pour a drink. What impact would this have on you? It would provide you the ability to get a drink when you want or need it. It would provide pride and self-worth through achieving something, and it would provide opportunities to gain praise and feedback from those you care about. The impact goes much wider than this. Learning some core skills could provide a foundation for more opportunities to gain skills, such as making small snacks, to managing hot food and drinks, further increasing independence and self-esteem.
- Imagine learning to drive. What impact would this have on you? It would provide the ability to access environments independently and allow you to travel further. Passing your test may result in praise from others and you may feel you have achieved a long-term goal. There may also be further impacts such as a career that involves driving or providing the ability to access leisure or work opportunities further away that you were unable to previously access.
- Imagine learning to manage your own money while still living at home with your family. What impact would this have on you? It would allow you to manage your own money and purchase items you choose, reducing your dependence on others. It may also provide the ability to save for your own home and instil key skills you will need for managing that household.

Imagine not having the opportunity to learn some of the skills highlighted above or any other skills you have gained. How would you feel if you were told you would not be given opportunities in the future to learn new skills?

For some people with intellectual disabilities, their opportunities for learning new skills are limited due to others feeling this may be too difficult for them or too difficult for the person supporting the teaching. There may be a belief that if the person has not learned skills by a certain age or stage, they never will. Danger and risk for the person with a disability can also be discussed when considering whether new skills should be taught (this is usually discussed when considering knives, hot appliances, accessing water, etc.). For some people with intellectual disabilities, opportunities to learn new skills have been given but due to it being at the wrong time, introduced incorrectly or taught without the right supports, the person has been unable to achieve the skill. These ways of thinking have resulted in a reluctance to try by those supporting the person. However, by providing opportunities to try new things at a pace that is right for the person and making adaptations to support their independence, new skills can be learned, and they can continue to achieve and flourish.

Enabling Capable Environments © Pavilion Publishing and Media Ltd and its licensors 2024.

Thinking space

We have shown that learning new skills is vital for immediate well-being and independence and to open opportunities for more skill development.

Imagine you had previously tried to learn a new skill (maybe driving a car) but you hadn't mastered it. At the time, you were going through a stressful time due to exams. You also didn't 'connect' with your instructor and felt his teaching style wasn't right for you. Now imagine others feel you don't have the ability to drive and it's risky to try it again. They feel that if you were going to learn, you would have picked up driving by now.

- How would you feel to be told you shouldn't be given another chance to learn?
- Would it be fair for others to disregard what you were dealing with at the time (exams) as a factor towards your ability to learn the skill?
- Would it be fair to think you were not able to learn the skill, rather than consider it being the way it was taught to you?

These questions should be our first considerations when discussing teaching new skills.

Life-long learning is key to continued growth and independence. When we support people with learning disabilities, there are some vital elements that will facilitate this:

- Opportunities to learn new skills must be targeted towards the person's preferences and abilities. We all want to be learning skills that are meaningful and important to us, not what others think we should be learning.
- Learning new skills should be fun. Help teach new skills linked to something fun (i.e. playing a new game, learning a musical instrument, etc.). You can also make the process of learning fun by incorporating things the person enjoys.
- Start small and move slowly.
- Use the communication methods the person prefers.

These are all key in building the person's confidence. Choice and control are key to independence and should be encouraged in all areas of a person's life. Those supporting the person should look for opportunities to encourage the person to take control.

Supporting someone to learn new skills can be difficult but it is crucial that the person is encouraged to select goals they want to achieve and that those that support them provide opportunities for them to learn these new skills. Having these goals written down for everyone involved is a good way to remember what the focus of support should be. In addition, it should be detailed how the person likes to be taught new skills and how they would like to be introduced to new tasks and experiences.

Personal care and health support

Personal Care and Health Support

In McGill *et al.*, (2020), the component of personal care and health support is outlined as follows:

> *'Carers are attentive to the individual's personal and healthcare needs, identifying pain / discomfort, enabling access to professional healthcare support where necessary and tactfully supporting compliance with healthcare treatments.'*

Why is this important?

It is identified by McGill *et al.*, (2020) that 'challenging behaviour is less likely when the individual is healthy and not in pain or discomfort'. They add that 'most people (with and without learning disabilities) attach the highest possible value to "good health" and want to receive personal support in a dignified way' (p6).

There is a risk, though, where it is seen that people are considered in good health if they are pain-free or not showing symptoms of poor health. This is not enough as it is well established that people with an intellectual disability often experience multiple barriers to accessing good health support to the extent that people with an intellectual disability:

- Die younger (up to 20 years) than others.
- Are more at risk from certain health conditions such as cancer and diabetes.
- Are more likely to be prescribed multiple medications for longer, sometimes with limited diagnosis to justify such medications (Doody & Bailey, 2017; Mencap, 2012).

Preventative healthcare for many people with intellectual disabilities relies on other people who may not fully understand the need for vigilance about healthcare

Enabling Capable Environments © Pavilion Publishing and Media Ltd and its licensors 2024.

or the additional complexity people with an intellectual disability face when trying to access healthcare.

Good health characteristics

Good health is an indicator of quality of life. In Schalock *et al.*, (2004), quality of life factors and domains are identified as physical well-being, emotional well-being and material well-being.

Emotional well-being is connected to feeling contented, a lack of stress and having a positive self-identity.

Physical well-being is associated with health and lifestyle.

Material well-being is associated with factors such as housing, somewhere safe to live and financial security to facilitate access to personal possessions.

We would suggest that there is a fourth domain to well-being, relational well-being, and have illustrated this as a figure below to represent **optimal well-being**.

Figure 3.1: Optimal well-being

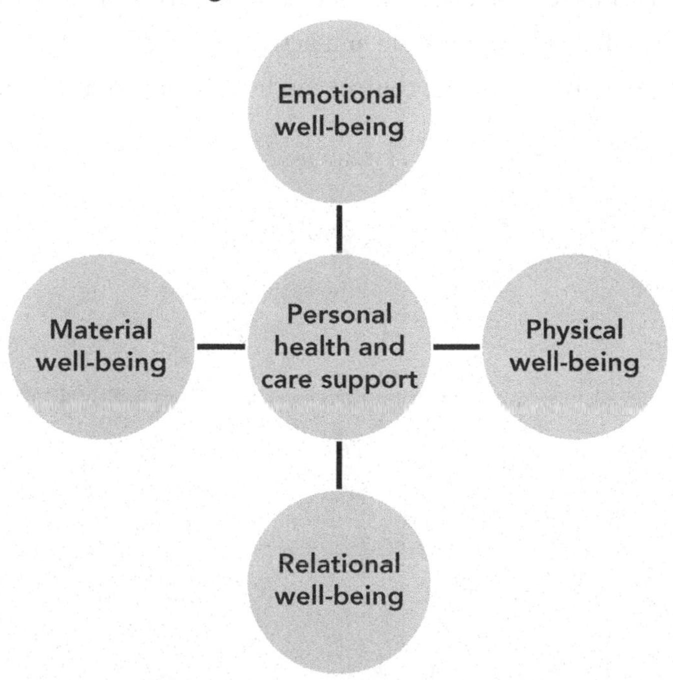

Relational well-being

People with an intellectual disability often experience loneliness and lack social connections. How does this relate to personal health? Recent research has identified that having a sense of belonging, the opportunity to engage in leisure activities, and having relationships that feel safe and empowering can have a significant positive impact on our physical and mental health and well-being.

Relational well-being is more than being symptom-free of illness; it is more active and dynamic. It is a more contextual approach to well-being, focusing on co-production and actively pursuing opportunities for optimum health and well-being. One model that can support relational well-being is Person-Centred Active Support (Chapter 7).

Person-Centred Active Support is based on evidence that:

- Engagement in activities and social relationships improves people's quality of life.
- Personal development is only possible when you participate in activities that broaden your experiences.
- Social relationships and inclusion depend on interacting with other people.
- Physical health depends on lifestyle and activity.
- Greater engagement, choice and control can lead to personal autonomy.

 Enabling Capable Environments © Pavilion Publishing and Media Ltd and its licensors 2024.

Thinking space

Using the table below, map out each of the components of optimum health with the individual and team you work with.

Component	Why is this important to the person you support?	What is currently working well?	What are the opportunities for development?
Emotional well-being			
Physical well-being			
Material well-being			
Relational well-being			

What is needed to promote optimum health?

Understanding of the legal framework. A need for a clear understanding of the legal frameworks to support decision-making and the process for decision-making where there is limited or lack of capacity.

Ensure better access is 'business as usual' not just something extra. There is some awareness of the need to make reasonable adjustments for people with an intellectual disability to access health care. Many health services have innovative resources raising awareness of what reasonable adjustments might be for example:

- Easy Read information sheets.
- The ability to make appointments at certain times of the day.
- Infographics and videos outlining certain procedures.

However, these resources have a limited impact if people with an intellectual disability or those who support them are not aware of them.

As a support team, it is important to recognise that changes in behaviour can be related to sensory, physical or mental health needs. Don't just rely on others to ensure routine health checks happen. Based on the work already done on the use of hospital passports, extend this to healthcare passports – healthcare does not just happen at a hospital.

Learn from research and inquiries. It is now established that there is a need for people with learning disabilities to receive their screenings at an earlier age. Those who support people with intellectual disabilities need to be more proactive in pursuing access to them.

Knowledge and understanding of the barriers to and enablers of optimum health is essential but more needs to be done to ensure mandatory training (where available) is focused on the impact of optimum health for people with an intellectual disability. As of yet, there is no overall solution, but we recommend that there is a need to 'bridge the gap' between what people know (learn in training) to what people do (actions to promote optimum health). We also recommend that those who support people with intellectual disabilities place a high priority on health through; accessing research and resources regarding health and learning disabilities, understanding the legal framework around choice and decision-making, enhancing their skills in Person-Centred Active Support, and remembering preventative healthcare is vital to well-being.

Conclusion

We have provided some practical examples of how the eight capable environments characteristics can be enhanced in everyday practice with people with learning disabilities. This information provides easy and simple ways to ensure capable environments can be established either at home, in your education setting or within supported services. Running through all the characteristics is the need for:

- Communication methods that meet the person's needs and preferences.
- Increasing choice and control in all areas of the person's life.
- Supporting engagement and participation at a pace and in a way that is right for the person.
- Listening to the person and understanding their needs, wishes and goals.
- Review practice to optimise learning and development opportunities.

 Enabling Capable Environments © Pavilion Publishing and Media Ltd and its licensors 2024.

Chapter 4: Sustaining capable environments – systems of support

In an interview in 2007, Jim Mansell said:

> *'It is not community care that is failing, but our ability to deploy the creativity, imagination, competence, commitment, and resources to make it a reality for people with complex needs such as challenging behaviour.'* (Ahmed, 2007)

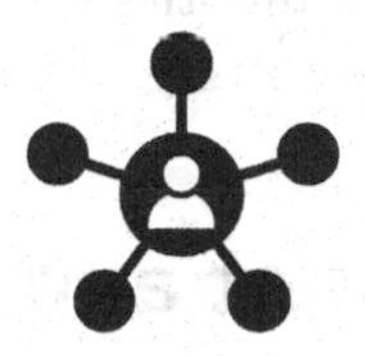

Chapter contents:

- Introduction
- Effective Management and Support
- Acceptable Physical Environments
- Mindful Skilled Carers
- Effective Organisational Context

Learning outcomes

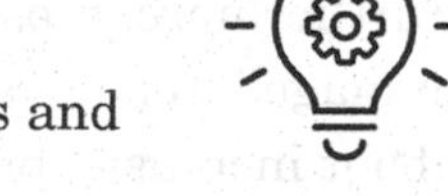

After reading this chapter and completing the suggested activities and reflection, the reader should be able to:

- Understand the leadership processes needed to sustain capable environments and personalised support.

- Have a critical understanding of the impact of physical environments on people's quality of life and well-being.
- Recognise the role of skilled, reflective staff in the provision of person-centred support.
- Appreciate the organisational contexts to supporting personalised supports and the impact of national policy and guidance.

Introduction

As discussed in previous chapters (Chapters 2 and 3), there are 12 characteristics that enable the development of a capable environment. Eight of these characteristics are areas that those working directly with the person can influence, change and adapt now (see Chapter 3). The remaining four characteristics require changes to the systems and processes that surround the person. This chapter will delve into the systems of support around a person that are required to sustain a capable environment. We will share examples from our experience and will provide practical examples of how the characteristics of capable environments can be enhanced in your home, educational setting, or support service.

Effective management and support

Effective management and support are vital to both creating and sustaining capable environments. McGill *et al* (2014; 2020) say:

> 'Challenging behaviour is less likely when carers are well-managed, led and supported. Most people (with and without learning disabilities) want to be confident that their carers (if they need them) are, themselves, well supported and can get help when they need it.' (p7)

Mansell (2007) identified that rather than relying on attempts to alter a person's behaviour, there is evidently a need to design services that promote a person's quality of life despite the intensity or frequency of behaviours that challenge. Furthermore, those supporting the person need to be trained, supported and managed in such a way that they can promote positive interactions that may bring about increased participation, independence, choice and inclusion within local communities.

Organisations are responsible for creating a climate in which staff know that the most important part of their job is providing effective person-centred support.

 Enabling Capable Environments © Pavilion Publishing and Media Ltd and its licensors 2024.

However, it is the frontline managers and supervisors who have the most focused and critical practice leadership role. Good leadership is required to ensure those supporting an individual work together as an effective team. The people providing support need to work consistently and to the agenda of the individuals they serve. Managers need to be able to support the development of staff knowledge and skills and to provide ongoing motivation and direction. Support staff or those responsible for providing direct support to individuals must be managed and supported by individuals with administrative competence and the skills to lead all aspects of capable practice. In this section, we will discuss key components of the managerial role that aim to improve the quality of life both for those supporting an individual and for the individuals supported within services.

Establishing and maintaining effective management and support

There are fundamental components that are required to create and maintain a focus on, and the delivery of, an enhanced quality of life and person-centred support as illustrated in Figure 4.1 below.

Figure 4.1: Effective management and support

Compassionate Leadership

Values

Shared Vision

Practice Leadership

Knowledge and Skills

Supervision

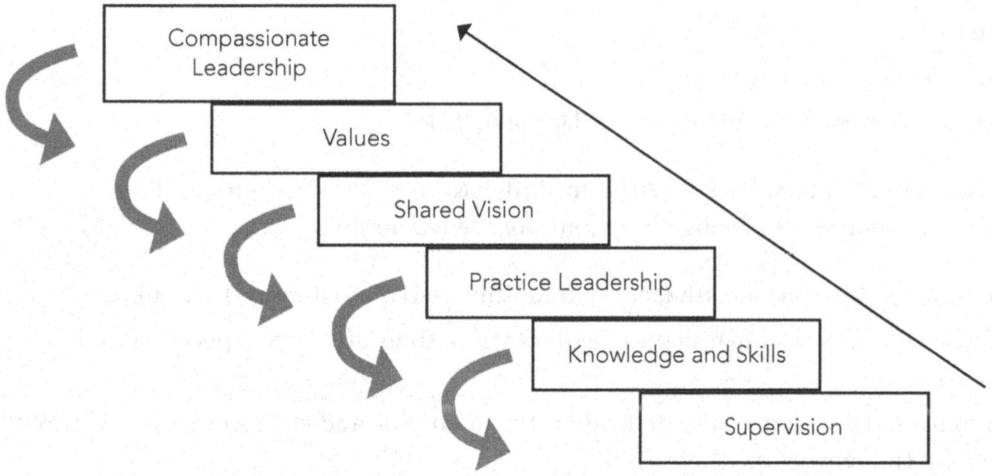

It is important as a leader to have a compassionate approach to your role. This approach will feed into the values, practice, knowledge, skills and support offered to those you lead. But effective leadership is not simply top-down, there needs to be a recognition of how staff perspectives and experiences influence our approach as managers.

Compassionate leadership

What is compassionate leadership?

Compassionate leadership is an approach to managing individuals, teams and organisations that prioritises the development of relationships. The approach focuses on leaders enhancing each member of their team's skills and knowledge to their full potential. This is achieved through leaders taking an empathetic perspective when engaging with their teams. They are encouraged to listen and try to understand challenges from their staff's point of view. Compassionate leaders support their teams in managing difficulties by supporting and enabling their teams to identify and deliver solutions collaboratively (Bailey & West, 2022).

The Impact of compassionate leadership

Work has shown that using this approach results in:

- Increased staff engagement.
- Increased staff motivation.
- Increased staff well-being.
- High-quality support.
- Reduced staff stress.
- Increased patient satisfaction.

(West, 2021; West *et al*, 2015; West & Dawson, 2012)

According to Atkins & Parker (2012, in Bailey & West, 2022), there are four behaviours required to facilitate compassionate leadership:

- *Attending*: Compassionate leaders take time to truly listen to their staff.
- *Understanding*: Compassionate leaders value their staff's perspectives and experiences.
- *Empathising*: Compassionate leaders try to understand staff's emotions without letting them overtake their own.
- *Helping*: Compassionate leaders offer support and resources to overcome barriers and challenges staff face so they can do their role to the best of their abilities.

Enabling Capable Environments © Pavilion Publishing and Media Ltd and its licensors 2024.

Values

Values can play a huge role in the provision that people receive from those who support them. Organisations and educational institutions are likely to have well-formed values that focus on the individual and their quality of life. A common issue that arises within these settings is the incongruence between these organisational values and the personal values of those employed by the organisation (this includes all levels of frontline and managerial support). This incompatibility of values can directly impact the types of support the person receives.

As a leader, it is important to recognise that everyone has different personal values, but these differences can greatly impact on the support provided. Furthermore, there must be a recognition that there is a need for organisational values to take precedence, ensuring they are embedded and delivered. Understanding what support is required to reconcile personal and professional values is critical to ensuring good person-centred support with a focus on improved quality of life for the individuals being cared for.

Shared vision

Quillam *et al.* (2017) identified that carers can feel powerless, disregarded, and disconnected in everyday practice. Although they agree with the values of inclusion and participation in general, some staff find it difficult to accept that these can be applied to the people they work with (Bigby *et al.*, 2009). It is therefore critical that the manager is able to communicate a shared vision of what the organisation wants to create. Shifting the culture from a focus on reducing challenging behaviour to a focus on quality of life needs strong leadership and teamwork. It requires a robust process that supports the implementation of those values by establishing what this means in everyday practice. This book provides an example of such an approach, and the processes required to imbed and maintain this.

Practice leadership

For leaders to deliver effective support they must consider the key messages staff get from their organisation and managers, as this guides their practice. From our experience, the common messages that tend to be communicated to staff across services centre on inspections, reports, audits and paperwork. Much of this focuses on what is *not being done well* rather than telling people what is working and supporting them to develop better practice telling people what they can do. These

Enabling Capable Environments © Pavilion Publishing and Media Ltd and its licensors 2024.

messages (on what is not being done well) tend to prioritise systems and processes rather than people's quality of life. As discussed throughout this book, ensuring people have a good life should be the central component of any service, educational setting or organisation.

In Chapter 6, we speak more specifically about practice leadership, in terms of how leaders can focus on building a staff team's skills and practice. However, as a general concept, practice leadership must be embedded in every area of a manager's role if they hope to facilitate a focus on quality of life rather than one of administration and compliance.

Skills for Care identify a manager's role as 'supporting the team's development into an effective and motivated group with person-centred care at the heart of what they do. [Managers] need to be aware of what learning the team needs to build upon their strengths and work towards eliminating their weaknesses' (Skills for Care, 2022). It should be noted that the responsibility for adopting an ethos of quality-of-life improvement does not and should not rest solely with a manager. The culture and values of an organisation must be aligned with this ethos.

Knowledge and skills

The Royal College of Psychiatry discuss in their 2007 paper, 'Challenging behaviour: a unified approach', that staff require foundational training before requiring more specialist input. They describe this support as fundamental and integral to all work with people with intellectual disabilities. This includes an understanding of person-centred approaches, psychological and/or behavioural interventions, signs and symptoms of mental illness, and values and principles of understanding and supporting people whose behaviour is described as challenging.

Further, the report states that staff teams should not be looking for quick solutions to what may be lifelong patterns. They need to be trained, supported and managed in such a way that they can promote positive interactions that may bring about increased participation, independence, choice and inclusion within local communities.

Supervision

Effective supervision benefits employees, managers and, most importantly, the people they support. It is a process of providing active support to staff, helping

 Enabling Capable Environments © Pavilion Publishing and Media Ltd and its licensors 2024.

them develop the skills, knowledge and understanding they need to improve their practice, and supporting the ongoing improvement of quality in our schools and services to ensure those they support have the opportunity to live the life they choose. The importance of supervision and reflective practice has been highlighted in several serious case reviews such as the Victoria Climbie Inquiry and the Winterbourne View serious case review.

Organisations have a legal duty to provide supervision for all their staff. This duty is reflected in the Health and Safety at Work Act (1974) as well as education and health and social care legislation. The main functions of professional supervision are widely recognised as educational, managerial and supportive.

One model of supervision that is used within organisations is reflective supervision. This is a two-way process that supports, develops, enables and maintains good practice and an individual's personal and professional development. Supervision provides an opportunity for discussion about everyday experiences and for both the supervisor and supervisee to learn from these experiences. Reflection and reflective practice are vital aspects of learning and development and should be recognised as such.

Thinking space

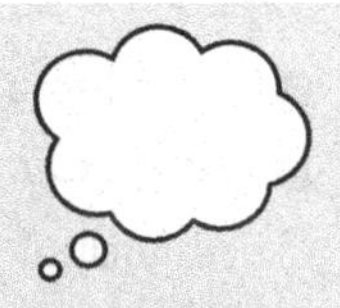

A mediator analysis is used to highlight the strengths and needs of a staff team to identify what support is required by the managers to enable and ensure better person-centred support.

Below is an example of a completed needs section of a mediator analysis conducted within a service supporting people with an intellectual disability and behaviour that challenges. This example identifies that:

- Supervision and reflective practice are infrequent.
- Some staff do not engage appropriately with Finn and leave him on his own for extended periods of time believing that this is what Finn wants.
- Some staff do not understand that Finn's behaviour serves a purpose and communicates a need.
- Newer staff do not have experience of working with people who display challenging behaviour.
- New staff require significant support and management when first working with Finn.

- Team Leaders are focused on several different duties which makes the implementation of PBS plans and strategies difficult.
- There can be inconsistencies in the support Finn receives depending on the experience of the staff member.
- Finn's community participation is inconsistent due to the views that staff have regarding his challenging behaviour and concerns over how to manage this.
- The service experiences high staff turnover.
- Staff work extra shifts leading to burnout and people being unwell.
- The service uses a high number of agency staff leading to inconsistency in support.
- Staff do not receive regular breaks during their shifts.
- There are no regular key team or team meetings.
- Staff also support several other individuals who display challenging behaviour.

Based on this example and what has been discussed in this section, take some time to think about what support, as a manager, you could offer to this staff team to address the issues highlighted within the mediator analysis. It may help to group the areas under the following headings:

- Knowledge and Skills – What type of training might the team require?
- Values – Are the values of the staff team compatible with the wishes of the individual and organisation? If not, how can you reconcile these?
- Supervision – Are staff receiving this? If not, how and when can this be introduced?
- Shared vision – Is there a shared vision? Do staff know what to do to work towards this vision? Do they have the practical skills?
- Practice leadership – Are leaders coaching and mentoring? If not, how could this be established and maintained?

Acceptable physical environments

McGill *et al*. (2020) say, 'Challenging behaviour is less likely in the absence of environmental "pollutants" (e.g. excessive noise). Most people (with and without learning disabilities) want to live and work in safe, attractive environments where they feel at home' (p6).

 Enabling Capable Environments © Pavilion Publishing and Media Ltd and its licensors 2024.

It will not be surprising to hear that the physical environment in which people live, is a critical factor in their well-being and quality of life. When people live and are supported in environments that are incompatible with their needs, their quality of life will likely be negatively affected. As we know, a reduced quality of life can result in behaviours that challenge. From our experience, rather than adapting the environment to meet the person's need, an expectation is placed on the individual to change or alter their responses, disregarding the external factors contributing to their distress. As discussed in Chapter 1, the links between environmental factors such as living conditions and social attitudes can have a significant impact on people's social inclusion and participation (Emerson & Hatton, 2014). We know that where people live and the values of those who provide their support will significantly influence their overall quality of life.

When discussing the requirement for people to live and be supported in acceptable physical environments, it is important to understand how people with intellectual disabilities have been treated and the types of physical environments they have had to endure in the past:

- In the early 1900s, people with intellectual disabilities were segregated in institutions and their identities were lost. They were hidden from society, spending their lives in settings far from their local communities with little to no contact with their families.
- In the 1970s, horrific stories of abuse within institutions were being highlighted by national newspapers, raising the profile of those with intellectual disabilities who had been hidden for so long, and exposing the horrendous conditions they were subjected to.
- This triggered the need for change, and from this the reform and de-institutionalisation model was developed and implemented. This often resulted in wards being divided to create smaller bedrooms, people having newer clothes and bed covers, and the improvement of food, but life was still the same for people with an intellectual disability.
- This began to change in the 1970s with two friends Jim Mansell and Alan Duncan. Jim was a university student who volunteered at Ely Hospital in Cardiff and Alan was a young man who lived in the hospital.

Their friendship and the experiences they had drove change for people with intellectual disabilities. This has been depicted in a 2023 musical called Housemates, which was launched at the Sherman Theatre in Cathays. The musical portrays what life was like for people living in such a setting. It shows how they

Enabling Capable Environments © Pavilion Publishing and Media Ltd and its licensors 2024.

were isolated from their communities, lived in overcrowded conditions, did not have their own clothes, and were ill-treated. Jim was appalled by the conditions Alan and others were exposed to. He and his fellow flatmates believed change was needed and decided to share their house with five people from Ely Hospital. This became the blueprint for supported living today. The play shows how Alan and other people's lives were transformed by living in a regular house and having the opportunity to participate in their community. Alan achieved his dream of playing in a band and Jim continued to have a leading role in the UK's closure of such institutions (hospitals). Jim's work and research continued to show that, with the right environment and the right support, people could be living exceptionally good lives.

Policy developments in *The Same As You* (2000), *Valuing People* (2001) and *Valuing People Now* (2009) made further changes and brought a greater focus on supporting people with an intellectual disability to live independently in the community. This brought hope that we would see a shift away from housing people in residential care homes and nursing homes, and towards supported housing and independent living models. Although this was noted as a positive step, the *Mansell Report* (2007) identified that the rate of progress had not been as hoped. Mansell noted that 'the failure to develop appropriate services has led to an increase in the use of placements which are expensive, away from the person's home and not necessarily of good quality' (Mansell, 2007, pg.ii).

Person-specific physical environments

It became clear that moving people out of hospitals and into homes that were not tailored to the person's needs was causing distress for people with an intellectual disability as well as their families and loved ones. Furthermore, it did not result in an increased quality of life and independence.

Heller (2002) conducted a literature review of the impact of residential settings which looked at identifying the key features associated with positive outcomes for people with an intellectual disability. These areas identified were:

- Homelike architectural features.
- Use of active support by staff.
- Use of assistive technology to facilitate independence.

Enabling Capable Environments © Pavilion Publishing and Media Ltd and its licensors 2024.

- Organisational policies promoting individualisation and person-centred planning.

Through our own clinical experience of supporting individuals in community and residential settings, we would also highlight the individual sensory needs as an important factor to consider when creating environments that aim to produce positive outcomes.

We will now look at each of these areas, considering their individual and collective importance in providing acceptable physical environments.

Homelike features

When we think of our own homes, it will conjure certain words such as, safe, secure, warm and cosy. What this means to each person is different (i.e. warm and darker colours versus lighter or white colours, ornaments versus a minimalist aesthetic, bright lighting versus low lighting, pattern prints versus block colours), but critical to this is the need for the environment to meet our individual preferences.

For a home to be considered as such, it must look and feel like a home to that person. It may be that people with higher support needs may require adaptations to the place in which they live i.e. tougher furniture, secured external doors, or less visual or acoustic stimuli, but this doesn't mean that the environment in which they live should be sterile. It should be 'homely' based on their preferences, and features such as décor, colour and light can have a huge impact on how comfortable, safe and secure people feel in their homes. For many people with an intellectual disability, the ability to live in their own homes is dependent on support from others and it is essential that their homes are not treated as workplaces in which work-related paraphernalia dominate any spaces.

It is important to consider the person's ability to access the people and places that are important to them. Living far away from family and friends isn't beneficial to the person if they would enjoy regular contact, visits and outings with them. Neither would securing a home in a busy city centre, if the person enjoys a slower and quieter pace of life. The reverse is also the case for those living in a rural

Enabling Capable Environments © Pavilion Publishing and Media Ltd and its licensors 2024.

community when they enjoy frequent access to leisure and recreational activities such as cinemas, clubs and shopping centres. Access to public transport and convenient travel to the things the person enjoys is essential for ensuring a home meets that person's needs.

In addition, a person's home should meet their physical needs. If loud noises are a concern, living near busy roads or a school shouldn't be considered. If a person uses a wheelchair, doors should be wider to ensure the person can move around their home without requiring support, and fittings should be lowered to their level to ensure they can access their amenities.

Thinking space

Think about your home. Imagine you were unable to decide the types of furniture, the décor, the lighting, etc. What if other people also chose who you lived with and where?

How would this make you feel?

There are many ways to gather information on a person's wishes regarding their home. You can:

- Verbally ask the person what want from their home. The person may verbally respond, they may write this down, or they may nod/shake their head to indicate their preferences.
- Show pictures or pictorial symbols, asking the person to select their preferences. The person may point to preferences or remove items they do not want in their home.
- Use samples and tester paints. The person will have the opportunity to see how these items look and may be able to select their preferences based on this.

Many simple changes can be made to a person's home to make them feel safe and comfortable (lighting, décor, furnishings). By gathering the person's views, many changes can be made to their homes quickly. Some factors may be more difficult to change (the location of the home, whom they live with, and costly changes to the property, for example) but this does not mean these considerations should be disregarded. There should continue to be a focus and discussion about the person's wishes and an active effort to pursue those changes. Those who support the person

 Enabling Capable Environments © Pavilion Publishing and Media Ltd and its licensors 2024.

should work collaboratively with all partners to advocate for them and to ensure their wishes regarding their preferences for their home are met.

Use of person-centred active support

In Chapter 7, we discuss the importance of providing person-centred active support (PCAS) as a key component in improving quality of life. But how does the physical environment impact the implementation of this approach?

Consider how accessible the environment is in allowing people to engage and participate in activities and pastimes, and offering them the opportunity to learn and build skills. Simple adaptations to the environment could support the person's ability to access the space safely (see Chapter 7).

Access to the items we need and enjoy is critical to our quality of life. Where a person's home is located is also critical to the ability to implement PCAS. Access to the local amenities that are important to the person is key to enhancing engagement, participation, and independence. Ensuring the person is close to these or that there are adequate travel links is essential. Where there are limitations to access, perhaps due to a clear risk, these risk factors should be regularly reviewed, and the use of blanket restrictions should never be used.

To ensure an environment can facilitate PCAS, time should be taken to consider the person's preferences and whether the home allows for them. If it does not, an active effort should be made to implement adaptations to support the individual's preferences and freedoms within their own home.

Enabling Capable Environments © Pavilion Publishing and Media Ltd and its licensors 2024.

Thinking space

Think about someone you know or support who has an intellectual disability. Consider the environment they live, work or study in:

- Are there any restrictions placed on them?
- If so, how do these restrictions impact the person's ability to access the things that are important to them?
- Do the restrictions limit the person's ability to engage, participate or enhance their independence?

If the answer is yes to the questions above, ask yourself:

- Is there a valid justification for these restrictions? (i.e., risk, safety, etc.)
  - Is there a clear plan to address the risks therefore making the use of restrictive practices unnessary?
- Are restrictions implemented with everyone, without consideration of individual needs?
  - What supports need to be implemented to change a culture that facilitates blanket restrictions?
- Is there a culture that promotes engagement and participation for people with an intellectual disability?
  - What support does the team need to maximise opportunities to enhance and improve people's quality of life?

Based on your answers above, it is essential to discuss this with a manager, head teacher, family member etc. to identify where restrictions can be removed or if adaptations can be made to limit the restrictions and increase quality of life for the individual.

Use of assistive technology to facilitate independence

The physical environment should include technology and equipment that allows someone to be as independent and in control of their life as possible:

 Enabling Capable Environments © Pavilion Publishing and Media Ltd and its licensors 2024.

- Specific communication technology may allow someone to navigate their way around their home independently i.e. signs or symbols on doors or cupboards to allow the person to understand what each room is and where things are kept.
- Colours and reflective strips may support a person with visual impairment to navigate their home independently.
- Technology within the home can allow people to keep in contact with family or friends (phones, computers, electronic tablets, etc.).
- Smart technology in the home allows the use of verbal language to make notes, reminders, or seek answers to questions (i.e. Amazon Alexa, Amazon Echo, Google Home, etc.).
- The use of adaptive equipment can allow people to have more privacy and dignity in their personal care routines such as privacy screens, walk-in showers or baths, plugs that automatically open when the water level is reached, etc.
- Alert systems can support a person's independence if they can call support when required, such as alarm systems the user can activate, sensors that detect falls, water overflows, seizure activity, etc.

Thinking space

Think about someone you support. Are there any assistive technologies that could be implemented in their home, classroom or day centre to increase their independence?

- Who might you speak to in order to identify whether these would work and whether they can be implemented?
  - This may be the person, their family, staff teams, your manager, the head teacher, etc.
- How might you introduce a new technology?
  - Discussing this with the person and those closest to them will be important.
  - If you want to implement multiple technologies, it may be beneficial to start with one until it's established and then move on to the next, depending on the person's preference and needs.
  - It may be useful to consider introducing the new technology but continuing to provide the current support until the technology is established and the person is comfortable and confident with its use.

Organisational policies promoting individualisation and person-centred planning

You have likely heard the term 'home comforts'. This is a term we use when talking about things in our home that make us feel good or make us feel safe. These items are undeniably our own and we may seek them out to provide positive feelings. We decide what we like, what we don't like, what we need, and what we don't, to gain those feelings. This allows us to function in a space we have designed to optimise our quality of life.

If a service is truly focused on providing person-centred support, then the starting point is for the person themselves to identify what they want and need from a home. Individuals should influence their own homes to create environments that benefit their personal needs. This starts with what the person wants their home to look like, to how their home can facilitate their aspirations and independence. This can be achieved by using person-centred planning tools regularly to gather the person's views and support their wishes. We discuss person-centred planning in more detail in Chapter 1.

If an organisation values person-centred planning and sees a sustained change in how people's homes, workplaces, educational establishments, and recreational spaces are designed, there must be an organisational policy to support this. It is not enough to assert this as a priority; organisations need to ensure they actively facilitate, monitor and review processes if they want to achieve person-centred support.

 Enabling Capable Environments © Pavilion Publishing and Media Ltd and its licensors 2024.

Thinking space

If you work for an organisation, it is beneficial to access your policies and identify which policy supports person-centred planning. You may need to ask your manager which policy pertains to person-centred planning.

If you can identify the policy:

- It is important to update yourself on the expectations of the policy and ensure you are working in line with its requirements.
- It may be beneficial to discuss the policy with your manager and agree on how this can be taken forward for the person you support.

If you cannot access a policy:

- It is important to consider how you may raise this with senior management to ensure it is promoted across the organisation you work for.
- You may be able to raise this with your manager at supervision or discuss it at an employee forum.
- Some organisations have ways to suggest improvements through online or physical request boxes.

Sensory considerations

Research tells us that differences in processing sensory information can result in motor praxis, attention difficulties, behavioural problems, increased anxiety, difficulties in performing routine daily living tasks, learning new skills, or coping in certain environments (Bundy et al., 2002). We all have different sensory sensitivities when it comes to our physical environment. They could be centred around colours, smells or noises. When supporting a person with an intellectual disability, you need to consider the appropriateness of the environment for an individual's sensory needs. Examples of this may be:

Noise levels. If a person is sensitive to loud sounds:

- Offer a quiet location for their home.

- Add soundproofing.
- Install triple-glazed windows.

If a person seeks loud noise:

- Offer a busy location for their home.
- Add technology that allows quick access to music.
- Soundproof the home to avoid disturbing neighbours.

Odours. Depending on whether the person seeks or avoids certain smells:

- Seek locations for their home beside or away from strong-smelling shops (i.e. soap shops, food establishments, etc.)
- Remove or add air fresheners and other scented items.
- Open or close windows and window vents.
- Install air conditioning to limit opening windows.

Temperature. People should be able to control the temperature of their homes, according to their preferences:

- Install air conditioning that the person can control.
- Install heating systems the person can control.

Tactile comfort. Taking into account the person's preferences:

- Purchase soft or hard furnishings.
- Provide different textured items.
- Remove items that cause distress.

Visual stimuli. Provide visual elements that align with the person's needs:

- Use block colours, whites, or patterns.
- Remove clutter or add ornaments depending on need.
- Install down-lighting if standard lights are distressing for the person.
- Add curtains and black-out blinds if they are sensitive to light.

It is essential to a person's quality of life that we understand their sensory needs and provide an environment that meets them. There are some ways to gather information on sensory needs:

Enabling Capable Environments © Pavilion Publishing and Media Ltd and its licensors 2024.

- Ask the person and they may be able to tell you their sensory likes and dislikes. If they communicate visually, they may be able to show you through pictures or symbols their sensory likes and dislikes.
- Ask those closest to the person. Speak to those who know the person well. Identify if they are aware of sensory sensitivities or environments that cause distress.
- Some allied health professionals, for example an occupational therapist, can complete sensory assessments and recommend strategies.
- Spend time with the person and try to identify situations or environments that cause distress and consider whether sensory needs may be the cause.

Thinking space

Now that we have discussed some of the key areas of focus in identifying acceptable physical environments, consider the following questions (which are applicable in most settings):

- Does your organisation adopt a person-centred approach to identifying acceptable physical environments for individuals requiring support?
- Think about someone you provide support to. Does the environment in which they live, work or study provide opportunities for them to actively engage in their life? i.e. are items required for learning new skills available, and does the person have access to all areas of the environment?
- Finally, would you describe the environment that they live in as 'homely'?

Mindful skilled carers

McGill *et al.* (2020) describe the component of mindful skilled staff as follows:

> 'Carers understand the general causes of challenging behaviour and the specific influences on the individual's behaviour. They draw on the expert knowledge of the individual's family and friends to improve their understanding. They reflect on and adjust their support to prevent and quickly identify circumstances that may provoke challenging behaviour.'

When working with individuals who engage in behaviours that challenge, you must be knowledgeable and skilled in doing so. This encompasses many areas of knowledge and skills, including:

- Knowledge about intellectual disability and the individual's specific diagnosis.
- How intellectual disability and a specific diagnosis impact the person and those around them.
- Strategies for supporting people with intellectual disabilities to engage, participate and increase independence (see Chapter 7: Person-centred active support).
- An understanding of why behaviours that challenge occur (see Chapter 9: Person-Centred approaches to understanding behaviours that challenge).
- Knowledge of the factors that specifically influence the person's behaviours described as challenging (see Chapter 10: Multi-elemental behaviour support plan).
- Specific strategies for responding to challenging situations safely and rapidly (see Chapter 11: The role of resolution strategies).
- Skills in coping with work demands and behaviours that challenge.

Understanding intellectual disability and co-existing health needs

Those supporting individuals with an intellectual disability and other diagnoses must understand what impact an individual's diagnosis has on the person and those around them. By understanding the person's diagnosis, you can understand how this affects processing, learning and sensory differences. This can help you understand the person better and provide the strategies and supports that may meet the person's needs. It is essential that those leading services, educational settings, or managing an individual's support, provide training and ongoing support on intellectual disability and, if applicable, any specific diagnoses.

Understanding behaviour

As stated by McGill et al. (2020), those who support individuals who engage in challenging behaviour must understand why behaviours form and are maintained (see Chapter 9). It is not enough to only understand why behaviours occur; staff teams should receive training in how to enhance a person's quality of life to address the factors that influence behaviours that challenge.

As well as general training in understanding behaviour, specific training should be provided around the factors that impact the person they support and the strategies that are effective in increasing their quality of life (see Chapter 9 and Chapter 10). They should also receive training in how to implement person-specific strategies

 Enabling Capable Environments © Pavilion Publishing and Media Ltd and its licensors 2024.

and safely and respectfully de-escalate challenging situations based on the person's needs.

If we hope to have skilled staff who can effectively support individuals and behaviours that challenge, organisations must provide training to increase knowledge among staff. A lack of knowledge results in inappropriate support, increased restrictions, decreased quality of life for those being supported, and dissatisfaction with the role within staff teams. Regular follow-up training sessions to support changes as well as continued knowledge-building are critical to sustaining good quality support.

Thinking space

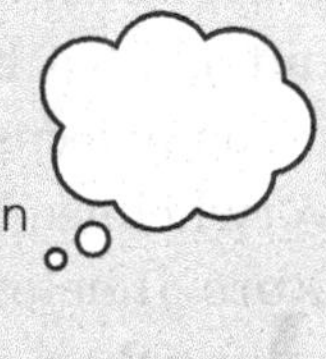

Consider the setting in which you work. Have you received the training and ongoing support you require to understand the needs of the person you support, as well as provide them with support to enhance their quality of life?

If not, what can you do to address this?

- You may need to speak to your manager to discuss how this can be provided.
- It may be worthwhile accessing respected websites and training providers to identify possible resources or training.
- Can you speak to family members, health professionals or social workers to gain more information?

Mindfulness

NHS guidance (2022) describes mindfulness as 'paying more attention to the present moment – to your own thoughts and feelings, and to the world around you'. The guidance recognises that we can often become caught up in being busy and going through the motions of day-to-day life without really paying attention to our thoughts and feelings in the present moment. Shapiro (2020) states that 'to be mindful' is to practice a way of being, a moment-by-moment gentle and nurturing awareness of our emotions and thoughts that can lead to breaking a cycle of negative thoughts. This is especially helpful when faced with stressful or difficult situations.

Enabling Capable Environments © Pavilion Publishing and Media Ltd and its licensors 2024.

Some examples of where this approach applies in practice settings were explored in studies that investigated if teaching mindfulness skills and techniques to staff alongside training in positive behaviour support would help reduce their stress and whether this would result in positive outcomes for the person being supported (Singh *et al.*, 2009; 2020). Singh's 12-session mindfulness decreased the number of incidents, staff interacted more positively with individuals, were more compassionate, reported being less stressed, and there was a reduction in the use of as-required emergency medication and physical restraint.

This method has been replicated on several occasions and has shown that mindfulness practice changes the interactions between those who provide support to individuals who engage in behaviours that challenge (including family, paid staff and teachers) and the people they support. It enables those supporting the person to focus more on what people need and want in the present and to not be overwhelmed by what has happened in the past or pre-empt challenges in the future. It helps to do this by changing the person's relationship with their thoughts, making them more aware of them, and helping them to understand that their thoughts are not reality.

Considering whether to, or how to, become mindful can be daunting. It can feel like a huge challenge and a move away from your usual ways of thinking and feeling, but as discussed earlier, the impacts on both you and the people you support can be significant. Below are some practical tips that can support a mindful approach in everyday life.

Figure 4.2: A mindfulness approach

Mindfulness Approach

Practice regularly: Little and often is the key. Take moments throughout the day, for instance on a walk, while waiting for the kettle to boil, while on the bus, and pay attention - what can you hear, see, smell?

Acknowledge your thoughts and feelings: Mindfulness is not about forcing ideas out of your head but acknowledging them and focusing on the here and now.

Try new things: A different route to work, sitting somewhere different for lunch, visiting the library – subtle changes to our daily routines can help us focus on our surroundings.

Create space to be mindful in your day: Use team meetings and handovers to focus on what is important today, what will a good day look like and how you can make that happen.

Enabling Capable Environments © Pavilion Publishing and Media Ltd and its licensors 2024.

There are also some practical resources that support your journey to a more mindful approach.

Practical ideas to help

The wheel of awareness by Dr Dan Siegel is available online. It is an awareness practice tool with a focus on breathing.

Headspace has a website and app which has resources such as meditation sessions and tips for everyday living.

The 'body scan' is another exercise aimed at mindful meditation where you can feel more connected to your physical and emotional wellness, this is accessible online.

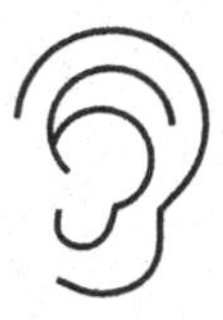

A helpful resource that can support mindfulness is the mindful listening tool for groups. Here, members of the group identify one thing they are stressed about and one thing they are looking forward to. The group work through a series of questions such as how to pay attention, cope with distractions and develop one's empathy.

Enabling Capable Environments © Pavilion Publishing and Media Ltd and its licensors 2024.

Thinking space

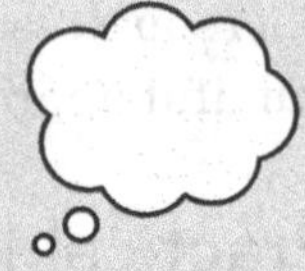

As we end this section, complete the table below and consider how mindfulness practices can become mindful actions in your day-to-day life.

Using the table, map the components of mindfulness and where it is working and where it can be developed.

Component	Why is this important to you?	What is currently working well?	What are the opportunities for development?
Reflecting on the value of what I do			
A space to learn and reflect on my skills			
A space to reflect and learn about what is important to the person I support			
A space to reflect and learn when things don't work out well			

Effective organisational context

McGill *et al.* (2020) say that to create an effective organisational context, 'Support provided by carers [must be] delivered and arranged within a broader understanding of challenging behaviour that recognises (among other things) the need to ensure safety and quality of care for both individuals and carers' (p7). They say this is essential because: 'Challenging behaviour is less likely when PBS informs the culture of families, service providers and service commissioners. Most people (with and without learning disabilities) want to receive evidence-based, well-governed support' (p7).

The original outline of this component discusses the need for practical organisational consideration within the context of challenging behaviour.

 Enabling Capable Environments © Pavilion Publishing and Media Ltd and its licensors 2024.

In our earlier work (Hume *et al.*, 2021), we discuss this in the context of quality of life and the quality of support for people with an intellectual disability.

To ensure that quality of life is prioritised and PBS is implemented well by those delivering direct support, organisations should ensure both quality of life and PBS are embedded within and influence the development of all systems and processes within their organisation:

- For instance, having only one standalone PBS policy that includes quality of life would not ensure that quality of life is prioritised and considered in every area, department and level of an organisation. PBS and prioritising quality of life need to influence all policies, every role, each system, and all levels of staff within an organisation or educational setting.
- A one-day PBS training session is beneficial but not sufficient to ensure PBS and quality of life are embedded in all aspects of an organisation and everyday practice. It is essential that all training delivered by an organisation is influenced by PBS. For instance, when training is delivered with a focus on support planning, quality of life and PBS should influence its direction and delivery.
- Prioritising PBS training and providing role-specific PBS training within an organisation is essential to ensuring personalised support becomes the responsibility of everyone in the organisation. This emphasises a clear focus on quality-of-life outcomes as the main function of the organisation.
- When developing job roles, the quality of life of the people receiving support should be emphasised and should influence all aspects of the job description. It is not enough for this to be prominent and influence direct support provision and direct line managers. All roles, including human resources, IT, payroll, etc. should understand how their role influences the quality of life of the people they serve.
- All levels of managers, particularly senior managers, members of the board and trustees should prioritise the quality of life of the people they support and place a focus on this in everything they do. Quality of life should be a set agenda point at all meetings, targets should be set, clearly defined, and regular monitoring should be implemented to ensure this is achieved.

There are examples of PBS implementation at all levels of an organisation that have resulted in positive outcomes for the organisation, its staff, and the people it serves. School-wide Positive Behaviour Support (SWPBS) combines behavioural interventions and organisational systems knowledge to create a culture that prioritises the success and achievements of students within educational settings

Enabling Capable Environments © Pavilion Publishing and Media Ltd and its licensors 2024.

(Horner, Sugai & Anderson, 2010). At the heart of SWPBS is a focus on the whole school as a unit, not the individual or a specific group. Assessment of the school unit and its needs is required and is followed by the implementation of supports (training, coaching, mentoring, and systems-change) to drive student success. What is critical in SWPBS is that everyone within the educational setting, at all levels and roles (i.e. janitorial staff, teachers, catering support) are provided the knowledge and the practical skills to achieve the agreed outcomes (student success) (Horner et al., 2010). A similar focus is being established within health and social care settings. Setting-Wide PBS was implemented in an adult social care setting with some evidence showing that improving the quality of social care through the implementation of Setting-Wide PBS may reduce and prevent behaviours that challenge (McGill et al, 2018).

What is needed for effective organisational context?

Based on our clinical work, we would suggest that a new model of support alone will not fix the deficits present in the models that organisations currently adopt. Instead, there must also be a focus on the context in which organisations function from an ecological model perspective.

Figure 4.3: Model of organisational context

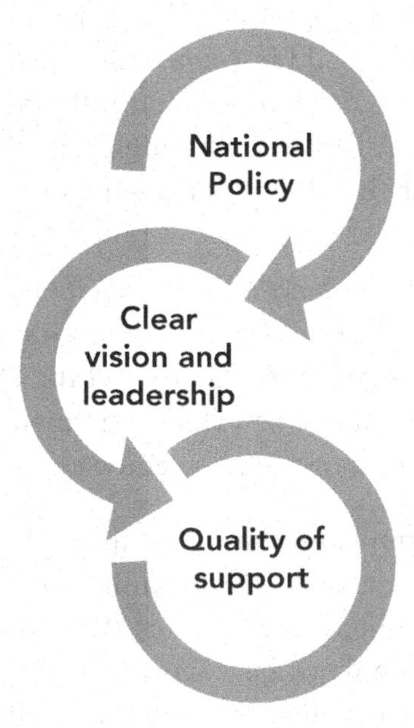

 Enabling Capable Environments © Pavilion Publishing and Media Ltd and its licensors 2024.

Organisations function in the context of national policy, and how this policy is implemented into reality requires clear leadership and vision. We know from the number of national enquiries that there are apparent issues at each of these levels in services for people with an intellectual disability. We draw upon a paper from Mansell et al. (2004) which is a call to action to move beyond person-centred planning to person-centred actions. We will apply this call to person-centred action to each domain in our 'model of organisation context' above.

National policy, clear vision and leadership, and quality of support

There is a need to quantify what is meant by quality of support and quality of life for people with an intellectual disability. A move away from counting the number of support plans written to understanding how they are implemented and whether they make any difference to the quality of people's lives is critical to this. Leadership will be the driver of this change and organisations can begin this process by focusing on their vision and value statements. Capturing what good practice looks like from the perspectives of people who use the service should guide the development of the vision and value statements.

This translation of an organisation's mission and values into their practical application should consider all service settings and should be a focus for review by:

- Families and people who use the service.
- Boards of trustees.
- Senior management teams.
- Quality monitoring teams etc.

Leading change

Leadership is central to implementing and influencing the quality of support a service provides. We discuss the role of practice leadership in more detail in Chapter 6. In this section, we outline Kotter's (1996) steps for leading change in organisations.

Kotter stresses the significant role of leadership in creating organisational change and promotes the role of leaders as enablers for change. We have adapted the components of these steps to reflect the need for leaders at all levels of the organisation to understand and align themselves, driving quality and change in services.

Enabling Capable Environments © Pavilion Publishing and Media Ltd and its licensors 2024.

Table 4.1: Process for leadership change

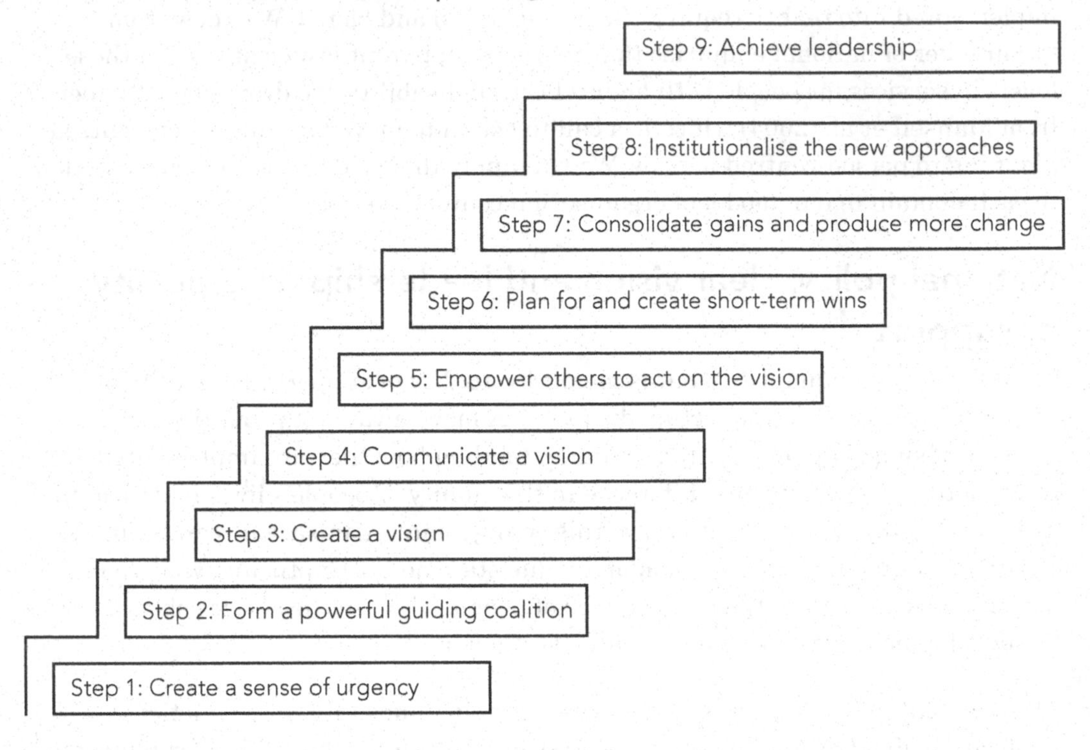

Within our pilot programme (Hume *et al*., 2021), we used Kotter's (1996) steps to change when developing and implementing capable environments.

Step one: Create a sense of urgency

It was critical to the process to ensure that the views of significant stakeholders were considered, particularly those who could influence change. This required understanding the perspectives of frontline staff, direct line managers, senior management, family members, and the individuals receiving support. It was important to know what they felt needed to change but also their vision for their roles in relation to the quality of life of those being supported.

Step two: Form a powerful guiding coalition

We then identified a group of key stakeholders who were keen to see change. This group met regularly to discuss the needs of the service, to organise and steer the development of the programme, and to monitor and review progress.

 Enabling Capable Environments © Pavilion Publishing and Media Ltd and its licensors 2024.

Step three: Create a vision

The guiding coalition met to decide the expectations of the programme with a focus on increasing the quality of life of those being supported within the service.

They established the expectations of each role to meet this goal, as well as the support needed to achieve the outcome of increasing the quality of life for the people living within the service.

Step four: Communicate the vision

The authors then organised and delivered regular meetings with all relevant stakeholders to communicate the progress of the programme, ensuring the vision (enhanced quality of life) remained prominent in everyone's minds.

Step five: Empower others to act on the vision

The authors met with trainee practice leaders regularly to identify barriers to the implementation of the programme. Critical to this process was the ability to support the trainees to enhance their skills in problem-solving and to develop solutions to barriers.

Step six: Plan for and create short-term wins

Data including Periodic Service Review (PSR) scores, quality-of-life measures, use of as-required emergency medication, etc. were gathered and reviewed collectively on a regular basis. This helped those leading and implementing the programme to see progress and support their continued investment. This process was supported by providing vouchers with monetary value to those implementing the programme well.

Step seven: Consolidate gains and produce more change

Regular review of data allowed the ability to make changes where required, showing stakeholders their views were appreciated and responded to.

Step eight: Institutionalise the new approaches

It was important to create a continuous improvement cycle to ensure that systems and processes support and sustain change and a continued vision of success. The introduction of the PSR allowed for ongoing review and maintenance of the programme.

Enabling Capable Environments © Pavilion Publishing and Media Ltd and its licensors 2024.

Conclusion

This chapter has provided information and examples of how changes to the systems and processes that surround a person can increase their quality of life and create and sustain a capable environment. This process requires a clear vision and strong leadership, an inherent drive to engage and listen to stakeholders (most importantly the person being supported), a collaborative approach to making changes, a commitment to ongoing monitoring, and a willingness to review regularly.

Enabling Capable Environments © Pavilion Publishing and Media Ltd and its licensors 2024.

Chapter 5: The Periodic Service Review: moving from an audit process to empowering personalised practices

'If we were sure what the perfect service looked like with perfect support, the process of evaluation would not be necessary.' (Capie, 1996)

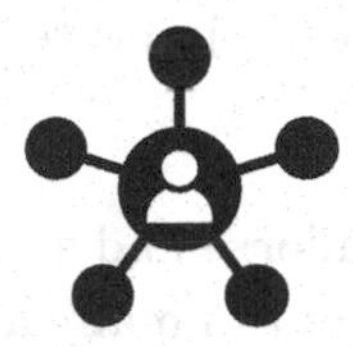

Chapter contents:

- Understanding the concept of quality.
- What is a Periodic Service Review (PSR)?
- How does a PSR enable quality support?
- Developing PSR standards.
- Implementing a PSR.
- Celebrating success and identifying opportunities.

Learning outcomes

After reading this chapter and completing the suggested activities and reflection, the reader should be able to:

- Recognise the key components of co-produced quality indicators.
- Identify how quality indicators are developed and appraised.
- Develop a co-produced PSR and a plan for its implementation and evaluation.

Introduction

The process of evaluation is a well-established method to inform evidence-based practice in service settings; however, this process is not always used routinely in person-centred practices (Mansell, 2007; Beadle-Brown *et al.*, 2014). While several regulatory bodies focus on standards and safety, such as the Care Quality Commission and the Health & Safety Executive, aspirations to meet such standards may not always guarantee that this is reflected in good practice in a service setting.

Services for people with a learning/intellectual disability have been required to comply with quality standards and regulations by governing bodies for several decades. Such standards are well-thought-out and designed to provide regulators with key indicators of what good quality service provision should entail. This type of regulation is typically measured by external reviewers using periodic assessments to ensure adherence to predefined quality standards or indicators. Methods of such assessment can include audits, self-report assessments, records reviews and observations or interviews. This process often relies on external assessors to judge if a service is compliant in its practices to indicate a satisfactory level of adherence to such standards.

The authors of this chapter fully endorse and support such external scrutiny and service reviews, and acknowledge that in many areas, such external assessment can illustrate some excellent examples of good practice. However, research and serious case reviews demonstrate that this process is not without risk if it is the sole means of judging quality. Serious case reviews have shown that, despite a service being in receipt of 'good' quality inspection reports or meeting the accreditation standards of a professional regulatory body, the abuse and neglect of people with an intellectual disability can still occur to the extent that staff and organisations become subject to criminal prosecutions, and people with an intellectual disability and their family can be traumatised by their experiences (The Challenging Behaviour Foundation, 2020).

Other research has demonstrated that there is insufficient attention to the quality of the support provided to people (Bigby & Beadle-Brown, 2016; Beadle-Brown *et al.*, 2017). This research suggests that the standards designed to monitor the quality of services provided may not reflect indicators of quality support from the experiences of people with an intellectual disability. A further consideration is that the evidence for external assessors is predominantly sourced from records and policies, paper-based tools, to determine compliance with standards rather than the explicit practices of support staff on a day-to-day basis.

Enabling Capable Environments © Pavilion Publishing and Media Ltd and its licensors 2024.

Finally, a further risk in this process is that external evaluation can be seen as an end goal, where, once endorsement or approval is given, people feel relieved and revert to 'business and usual' until the next inspection. In such scenarios, evaluation becomes a product whereby minimum standards are achieved when in fact it should be seen as a process that will create change and improvements for all participants.

This first section of the chapter will focus on those who deliver the service, as often this is an area overlooked in how we define and measure quality. The quality of support can be appraised or assessed in several ways, however, this section of the chapter will refer to two methods: a Capable Environments Appraisal (CEA) (Hume *et al.*, 2021) and the Active Support Measure (ASM) (Beadle-Brown *et al.*, 2015).

The second part of the chapter will then outline how to develop a Periodic Service Review (PSR) as a method of implementing and evaluating a co-produced quality assurance system that can be applied across multiple parts of the system of support. Such an approach can be viewed as a non-linear approach, which mitigates some of the risks of reliance on external scrutiny and has a more explicit focus on the impact of direct support practices and improvements to a person's quality of life.

Understanding the concept of quality

The quality of staff support begins with planning what and how this support should be delivered (Mansell & Beadle-Brown, 2012). Good mainstream practices need to be well developed and organised with a clear goal to improve the individual's quality of life. The use of external assessment of quality is an essential part of the governance and regulation of services, but as a singular approach, it is insufficient. Figure 5.1, below, depicts an example of how key drivers from national policy and legislation correctly influence adherence and reporting structures at a local policy level; however, research and serious case reviews reveal that these drivers can function in a compartmentalised way which is process-driven. For example, there can be various drivers and agendas that inform national policy, but they may not be developed in partnership with inspectorate services, leaving local policy developers to 'interpret' what may have been a well-intended incentive but has little impact on directly improving people's quality of life and can lead to negative outcomes for individuals in the name of 'following a policy'.

For support teams, the narrative about improving people's quality of life becomes confusing because they don't know what to do or how to do it.

Figure 5.1: A compartmentalised approach to quality

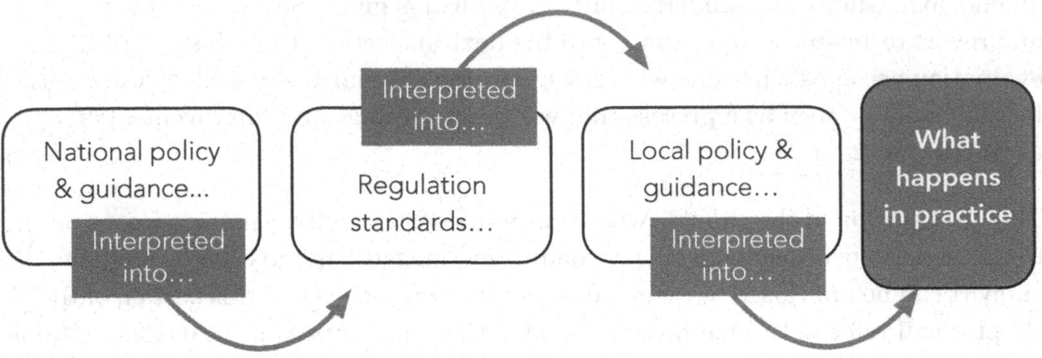

As an illustrative example:

- National policy: All children should have access to education.
- Inspectorate standards: All children should attend school for 80% of each term.
- Local policy: Parents will be fined if child attendance drops below 80%.
- Direct support: Family member must leave their employment to support their child at home.
- Individual practice: The school labels the child and family as non-compliant.

What is lacking is the knowledge among the people providing support of what to do **in practice** to ensure that they are providing quality support to enhance a person's quality of life, rather than just trying to interpret what they think policy requires of them.

 Enabling Capable Environments © Pavilion Publishing and Media Ltd and its licensors 2024.

Thinking space

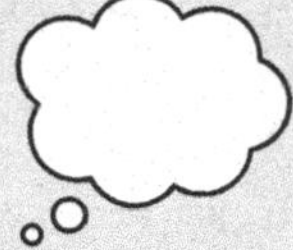

In many job descriptions there is a section referring to promoting choice and inclusion.

- Are you clear what that means in terms of what you do in practice, or is it something you must stop and think about?

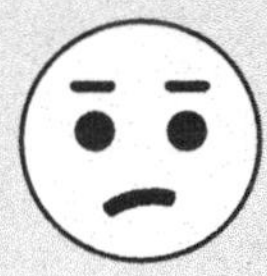

- What does that look like in your day-to-day role?
- Are there specific plans to show you the steps?
- Have you attended training to show you what that could look like?
- Is the topic of choice and inclusion discussed as part of your team meeting? Your supervisions?
- If promoting choice and inclusion is part of your day-to-day role, how do you know if you are doing it well?

Capie, as early as 1996, suggested the need for a more values-based process to inform the evaluation of good practice and stated that:

'We evaluate services because we want providers, service users, and families looking together at what service users value, and if practices do not reflect such values, examining how the service can be improved to enhance the lives of individual consumers.' (p75)

In addition, Hume *et al*., (2021) would advocate an approach that is driven by values and the needs of the individual, which strives to enrich the quality of support provided and experienced (Figure 5.2).

Enabling Capable Environments © Pavilion Publishing and Media Ltd and its licensors 2024.

Figure 5.2: Enhanced approach to quality supports

Individual needs and preferences
Direct supports
Local service policy
Inspectorate standards
National policy & guidance

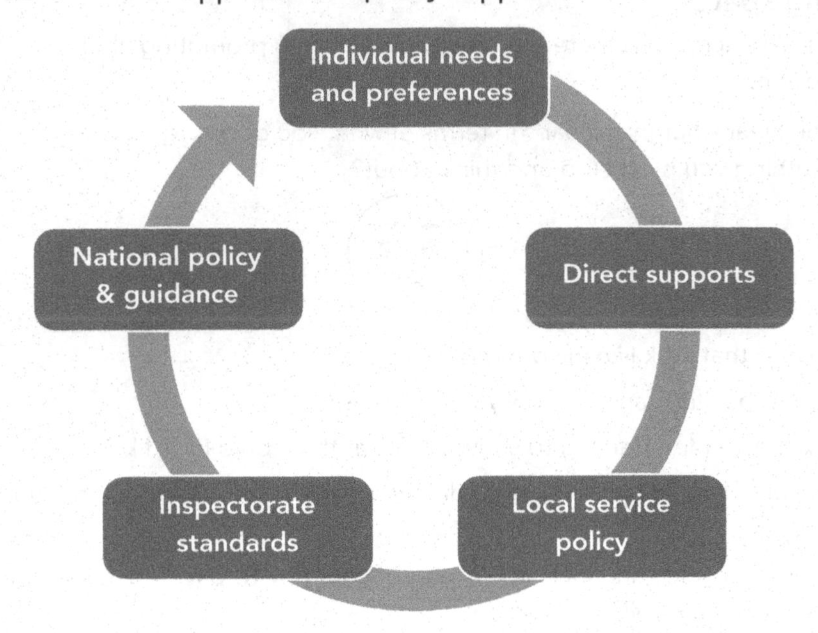

Thinking space

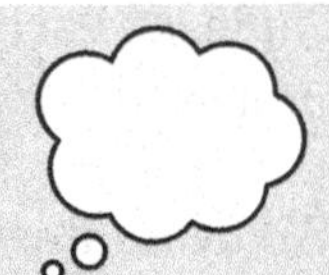

The discussion above looks at the relationship between quality of services and quality of support.

1. List the ways in which you know you provide good support on a day-to-day basis.
2. How does the support you provide enhance an individual's quality of life?
3. Where do you get feedback about the quality of support you provide?

Quality of support

We have established that the quality of a service as decided by external scrutiny is insufficient to ensure people experience a good quality of life. The quality of support provided is a more robust indicator that people experience support in a way that is meaningful to them and their support needs.

Quality support is a **dynamic process** (Figure 5.3) and, as such, helps to develop, implement and evaluate such supports. There are several frameworks

 Enabling Capable Environments © Pavilion Publishing and Media Ltd and its licensors 2024.

and approaches discussed elsewhere in this book (see Chapter 7, Chapter 9 and Chapter 6) that facilitate good quality support. However, all person-centred approaches need to become dynamic, person-centred actions in day-to-day practice.

Figure 5.3: Dynamic appraisal of quality support

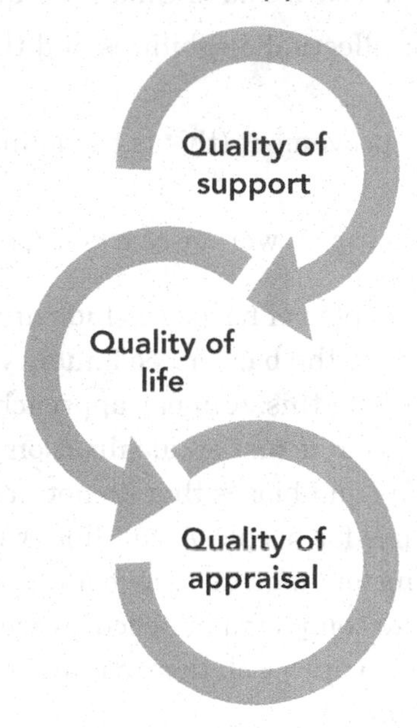

What do we mean by a dynamic process? Simply, it is a process which moves beyond just saying that someone has done something correctly. Instead, it is an active collaboration to identify the critical components of support and its ongoing development, implementation, and evaluation. All too often, support staff arrive at their roles unprepared for the day-to-day reality of trying to interpret assessments and support plans without clear support to understand the theory behind them nor the practical support to implement them. Help to implement quality support should be experienced as a developmental-orientated activity, not as a task to be done. Practice leaders play a key role in facilitating this dynamic process, for example, implementing quality support requires mentoring, coaching and feedback as you practice (see Chapter 6).

Research by Topping *et al.* (2022) looked at the key factors that staff perceived as being necessary for good service quality. Of interest, many of their perceptions of good service quality stemmed from their ideas and beliefs about how the services they had worked for could be improved, and barriers to good service quality removed. This research showed five factors that describe the practices and characteristics staff believed to contribute to 'good service quality':

- Collaborative, hands-on leadership (we discuss this in Chapter 6).
- Well-planned services (we discuss this in Chapter 1 and Chapter 2).
- Respect for people with intellectual disabilities and their carers (we discuss this in Chapter 1).
- A culture of continuous improvement (this is the foundation of this PSR chapter).
- Professionalisation of the support worker role (see Chapter 1).

Topping *et al*. (2022) is an exemplar of how to include and validate a more collaborative approach to setting the bar for good quality support and identifying the standards (steps) to achieving this. A linear approach in which people are expected to simply follow the plan is just an idealisation of providing positive support, based on assumptions and biases that do not necessarily translate into positive quality of life outcomes for people. A non-linear model provides a better fit because it moves from viewing 'management' as being responsible for confirming or validating quality according to completed or specific targets being met. There are key indicators of a collaborative approach to providing quality support. As a team consider the following questions:

- Is the support I provide dynamic and evolving?
- Are written plans detailed and considered to be necessary by all the stakeholders? Does everybody agree and know what is required?
- Is there a system monitoring what is in place, celebrating achievement and knowing what is going on?
- Are we always reviewing and planning for the next step, setting the agenda for person-centred action?

What is a Periodic Service Review?

The Periodic Service Review (PSR), developed by La Vigna *et al* (1994), is a self-reporting process that supports quality assurance. It is essential to understand that this is not an audit or inspection procedure; instead, it is an appraisal with a focus on fully engaging in continuous quality improvement.

 Enabling Capable Environments © Pavilion Publishing and Media Ltd and its licensors 2024.

The drivers that influenced the development of PSRs originated from the field of organisational behaviour management (OBM), in which there is a strong emphasis that all organisation members have a shared role in generating ideas and solutions. Creating a culture of creative thinking leads to increased staff autonomy by developing a shared vision with the team. Recent research developments emphasise that leadership is no longer viewed as something done to employees by a formally appointed 'leader', but rather as a dynamic social process and a collective activity generated by the collaborative interactions of colleagues, and other stakeholders, working toward a shared goal.

The PSR is both a means to help teams assess the level of quality in the services they provide and a system to help improve that quality. The PSR system provides teams with a direct and precise view of the effectiveness of their service. This systematic, or periodic, visual feedback is based on their regular assessments of every aspect of the service that is considered essential. Moreover, this assessment can be directed to managers, individuals, teams, classrooms or the organisation. The primary means for the Periodic Service Review is a set of specific Quality Standards (process and outcome), each of which describes a particular dimension of the service and its measurement criteria.

How does a PSR enable quality supports?

Research reviews of person-centred approaches, such as person-centred planning, positive behaviour support and communication supports, frequently find a vital issue with implementation where people must follow a plan consistently.

This is referred to as implementation fidelity – which is doing something the way it was designed to be done. However, when plans do not work, staff are blamed for not implementing the plan correctly. This can lead to an impasse (Figure 5.4), which means people get stuck in a cycle of saying the plan doesn't/won't work, people stop following the plan, people get blamed for not following the plan, people then believe the plan is not working, and then quality support does not happen.

Enabling Capable Environments © Pavilion Publishing and Media Ltd and its licensors 2024.

Figure 5.4: The cycle of ad hoc support

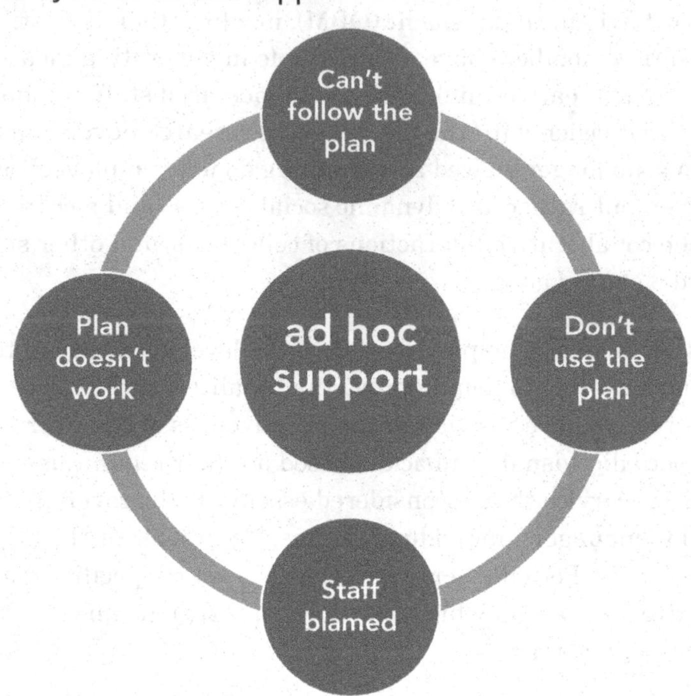

Keeping a narrow focus on implementation or following a plan for the sake of it, rather than thinking about the process and outcomes, can become something to tick off. This risks promoting an all-or-nothing attitude to the plan (the plan doesn't work, let's stop doing it). Instead, a PSR attempts to help teams/families/educators identify what can be done, it provides clarity and keeps a focus on good things about the plan and what steps to take to get there. It acknowledges that we are all developing our practices, and a PSR is a process to support this.

What needs to be considered in these situations are the following key questions:

- Is this plan suitable for our setting?
- Do people have the time and the training resources to do what is needed?
- What are the measures of success, and who determines these?
- Is the goal/plan realistic?
- How do we consider setting goals? Do we listen to people, or lift a process from a glossy website or copy someone else's plan?
- Are we blaming people, or are we listening and adjusting the plan accordingly?

 Enabling Capable Environments © Pavilion Publishing and Media Ltd and its licensors 2024.

Identifying standards

A PSR is a way of organising the steps of the plan (process) and what the plan should achieve (outcomes). These are called PSR standards. The overall aim of these standards is to improve the quality of the service, and the quality of support leading to quality-of-life outcomes.

Everyone should be involved

Trying to get engagement and buy-in before rolling out a vision or a plan puts a few people in charge and seeks compliance, it becomes a top-down model (see Figure 5.5 below), which does not promote the alignment of goals or plans that have meaningful outcomes for the individual or the support staff trying to implement them. It is so much richer and more meaningful to value relationships, and diverse perspectives and let ways evolve naturally.

Figure 5.5: Top-down model of compliance

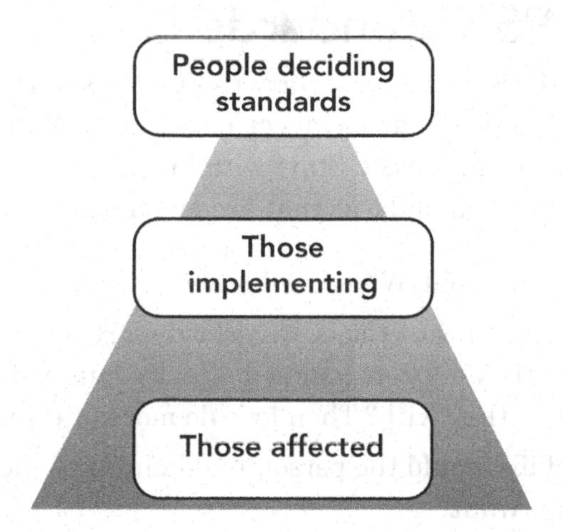

Enabling Capable Environments © Pavilion Publishing and Media Ltd and its licensors 2024.

Group Activity

As a team/family/classroom, use either the Capable Environment Appraisal (see Chapter 2 with details of how to use) or the Active Support Measure, and use your findings to begin your PSR. The template to write a standard for a PSR is provided below.

Some key points to remember:

- Start small – move slow – you do not need to do everything all at once, pick three or four standards to get you going (LaVigna *et al* 1994).
- Think about how often you will expect the standard to be implemented.
- Table 5.1, below, can be a helpful way to draft your standards in a way that is specific and measurable.

Developing PSR standards

One of the original authors of the PSR, Gary LaVigna, used the term 'start small, move slow' (LaVigna, 1994), and he means exactly that when thinking about developing and implementing a PSR. Start with just a couple of standards and build upon these. Start with standards that are meaningful, fun and functional.

- Meaningful to the individual. What would they prioritise?
- Fun for the individual. In workshops, we ask support teams to think about the last time the person they support laughed – really laughed out loud. What were they doing? Who were they with? Then let's do more of that.
- Functional. What skills would the person find helpful to them to meet their own needs whenever they want?
- It can be based upon an appraisal of current support such as the Capable Environment Appraisal, or a review of the quality of support such as the Active Support Measure.

After completing a review or appraisal, a process of summarising the findings and identifying priorities needs to take place (See Chapter 2 for more information on how to do this collaboratively). The conclusions drawn from this process then need to be transformed into PSR standards to support implementation and monitoring. To ensure consistent and quality support, there are some key elements that a PSR should focus on.

Enabling Capable Environments © Pavilion Publishing and Media Ltd and its licensors 2024.

These should be specific and functional to map progress and support which are indicators that good quality support is happening. By this, we mean there is clarity in what you are expected to do or see. It should also clearly illustrate the outcome (i.e. what should happen because of the action?).

A standard should:

- Emphasise what is essential to the person.
- Be realistic – has everyone agreed that it can be done and do they have the resources and support to do it?
- Have clear criteria – what, when, how and why.
- Be verifiable – how do you know it when you see it?

To ensure that everyone supports the implementation of PSR standards, we recommend the following:

- The monitoring of the standard is straightforward and relevant.
- Feedback on progress is readily available to everyone.
- Specific training is linked to each standard.

LaVigna *et al*. (1994) provide a template to develop individual standards for a PSR. An illustrative example is provided in Table 5.1, below.

This standard is based on a PSR developed by a family member who employs a staff support team.

What	Exactly WHAT support staff will to do in OBSERVABLE terms. *When Petra signs 'call' support staff will show Petra her photo friend books and ask, 'Who do you want to call?'* *When Petra points to a person in her photo friend book support staff will click on the iPad to call that person*
When	Specify exactly WHEN the action should be carried out. *Every time Petra signs 'call'.*

Who	Specify WHO is responsible for ensuring this plan is achieved. Everyone who provides support to Petra should ensure they are aware of how Petra indicates she would like to call someone. They are responsible for following the plan on a daily basis.
How	Specify HOW you will know the action has been carried out (e.g., direct observations, ability to answer questions on subject, ability to describe process in detail, record review) ■ A colleague directly observes this. ■ Daily diary records the Petra video called [NAME]. ■ [Insert name of friend] - says at a visit it was lovely to chat with Petra on a video call last Wednesday.

Implementing standards

The PSR should be user-driven rather than manager-mandated. Because the system is user-driven and each criterion is defined by the individual or team implementing it rather than by the organisation. The users of the system are measuring themselves against a set of tasks that they describe as being included in their role. This can also form the basis for ironing out inconsistencies between the individual/team view of what is expected and is a way to identify and celebrate good person-centred practices.

Areas to develop standards are, of course, specific to what your PSR is based on, for example, a Capable Environment Appraisal (see Chapter 2), a Multi-Element Behaviour Support Plan (see Chapter 10), and other person-centred framework such as the Active Support Measure (see Chapter 7). A simple example of a PSR standard that a practice leader might typically set for themselves is set out below:

 Enabling Capable Environments © Pavilion Publishing and Media Ltd and its licensors 2024.

Standard heading *Supervision meetings*
Process standard *Supervision meetings will be held once monthly on the third Friday of the month*
Outcome standards ■ Practice leader and support worker will attend the supervision meeting at 10am each third Friday of the month. ■ The practice leader will have completed three direct observations of practice prior to the supervision meeting. ■ A meeting agenda will be emailed a minimum of five working days before the meeting date. ■ A copy of meeting outcomes and actions will be sent to all within two working days of the meeting date.

Thinking space

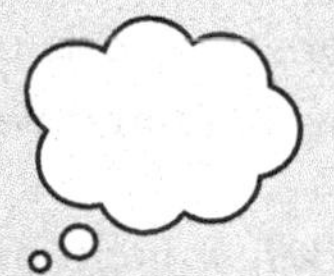

1. What influences what you do on a day-to-day basis? A support plan? Other people? The person you are supporting?
2. Using the table below write a standard about how you communicate with the individual you support.
3. Using the table below write a standard about how you should introduce an activity to the person you support.

Standard heading
Process standard
Outcome standards

Monitoring standards

Comparisons between the desired process and outcomes form the basis for individual data points. Each standard is allocated points, and these are either achieved when completed as stated or not achieved on this occasion but can be achieved in the future. During the review session, all points are added together and compared against the overall possible score that could have been achieved to produce a percentage score (i.e. total achieved score divided by overall possible score, times by 100). These individual data points are then combined and graphed over time. Teams can not only visually see improvements in their service/practices over time but can pinpoint what is working well and where the opportunities are for improvement. Visual feedback is a compelling motivator which gives us a level of motivation in our role that is seldom experienced. Such feedback should form part of team meetings, supervision and any other forums in which teams come together, for example, daily handovers. In keeping with the philosophy of how a PSR is developed (bottom-up approach), feedback, monitoring and development of future standards should also be generated by the direct team and the individual. Discussion about implementation of standards can be daily and we would recommend that the entire PSR is scored weekly and reported throughout the wider organisation.

Below is an example of how to plot a weekly PSR score using Excel. This format is easy to update and can be emailed to the team and a PDF printed to be placed somewhere it is visible to everyone.

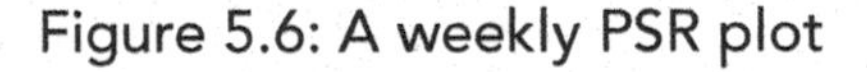

Figure 5.6: A weekly PSR plot

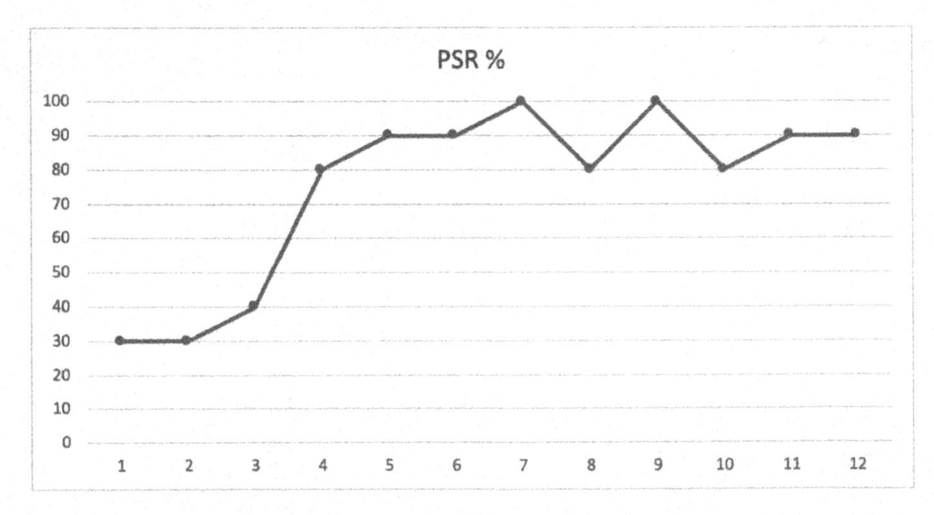

 Enabling Capable Environments © Pavilion Publishing and Media Ltd and its licensors 2024.

Implementing a PSR

Supporting a team to implement plans needs to be a comprehensive and ongoing process; writing a plan and assuming everyone can follow it is not sufficient. In their pilot programme, Hume *et al.* (2021) found that the evidence-based approach used in practice leadership is the most effective way to ensure plans are co-produced and co-evaluated. Further details on practice leadership can be found in Chapter 6 but the principles outlined by Mansell *et al.* (2004) include:

- **Focusing** all aspects of support on the quality of life of individuals and how well staff support this.
- **Allocating and organising** staff to deliver better support, when and how the people being supported need and want it.
- **Coaching** staff to deliver better support by spending time with them providing feedback and modelling good practice.
- **Reviewing** the quality of support provided by individual staff in regular one-to-one supervision and finding ways to help staff improve it.
- **Utilising regular team meetings** to review our effectiveness in supporting people to engage in meaningful activities and relationships and to find ways to improve.

A key focus of a practice leader is to help people move from being able to say what needs to be done (verbal competence) where they can describe what they should do and why, to doing it in practice (practice competence) where people do what is needed (LaVigna, 1994).

This form of scaffolding, from knowing to doing, fits with many of the components of practice leadership as outlined above. Typically, teams need support to move from reading a support plan. They need time to be spent with them, with the practice lead providing clarifying, coaching and providing feedback at each of the steps illustrated below.

Enabling Capable Environments © Pavilion Publishing and Media Ltd and its licensors 2024.

Figure 5.7: Scaffolding support plan competency (five tiers to competency) (Adapted from LaVigna, 1994)

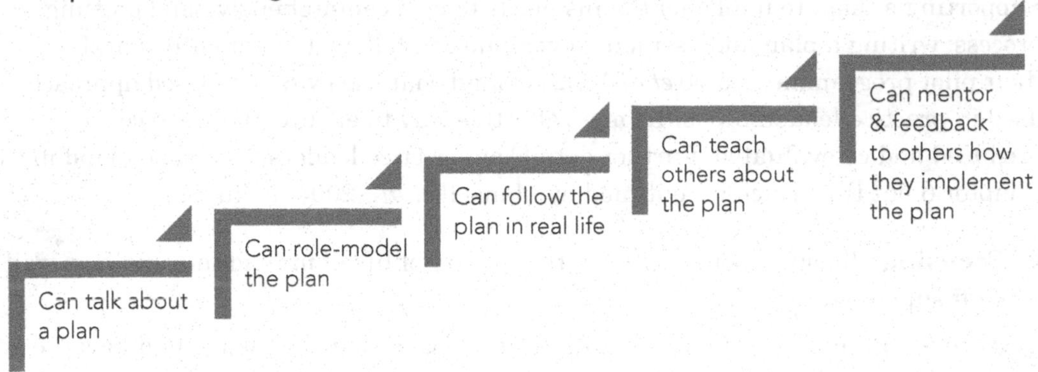

Celebrating success and identifying opportunities

The PSR and its standards are developed alongside the team implementing the plan. These standards are operationally defined and are reviewed at agreed intervals, usually weekly but no more than monthly, to identify how well the plan is being implemented (McClean & Grey, 2012). It is crucial that the score from this review is shared with staff, and it is preferable that the graph from the review is visual feedback (La Vigna *et al*., 1994; Hume *et al*., 2021).

Within the study by Hume *et al*. (2021), participants were supported to develop PSR standards for their focus person based on the ten capable environment components. The PSR focused on how to observe and identify whether a standard had been achieved. The participants were supported to complete the PSR weekly with a focus on permanent products and/or observations. They were encouraged to display graphic feedback showing changes, achievements, and further opportunities within offices that staff would use frequently. In the development of the PSR with this team, the idea of ten a day became a focus (ten a day was a nod to the idea that ten pieces of fruit or vegetables a day are good for you) and they scored themselves not in number but a hierarchy of vegetables or fruit, so, for example, a Brussel sprout was two where a dragon fruit scored ten – whatever it takes to motivate a team should be considered, even if its vegetables!

This was used to identify areas/components that required further support. The PSR was an essential element of the framework and outcome measurements. These

 Enabling Capable Environments © Pavilion Publishing and Media Ltd and its licensors 2024.

measures were used to show whether the key components of capable environments were being met in practice.

Figure 5.8: 'Ten a day' PSR score and number of incidents

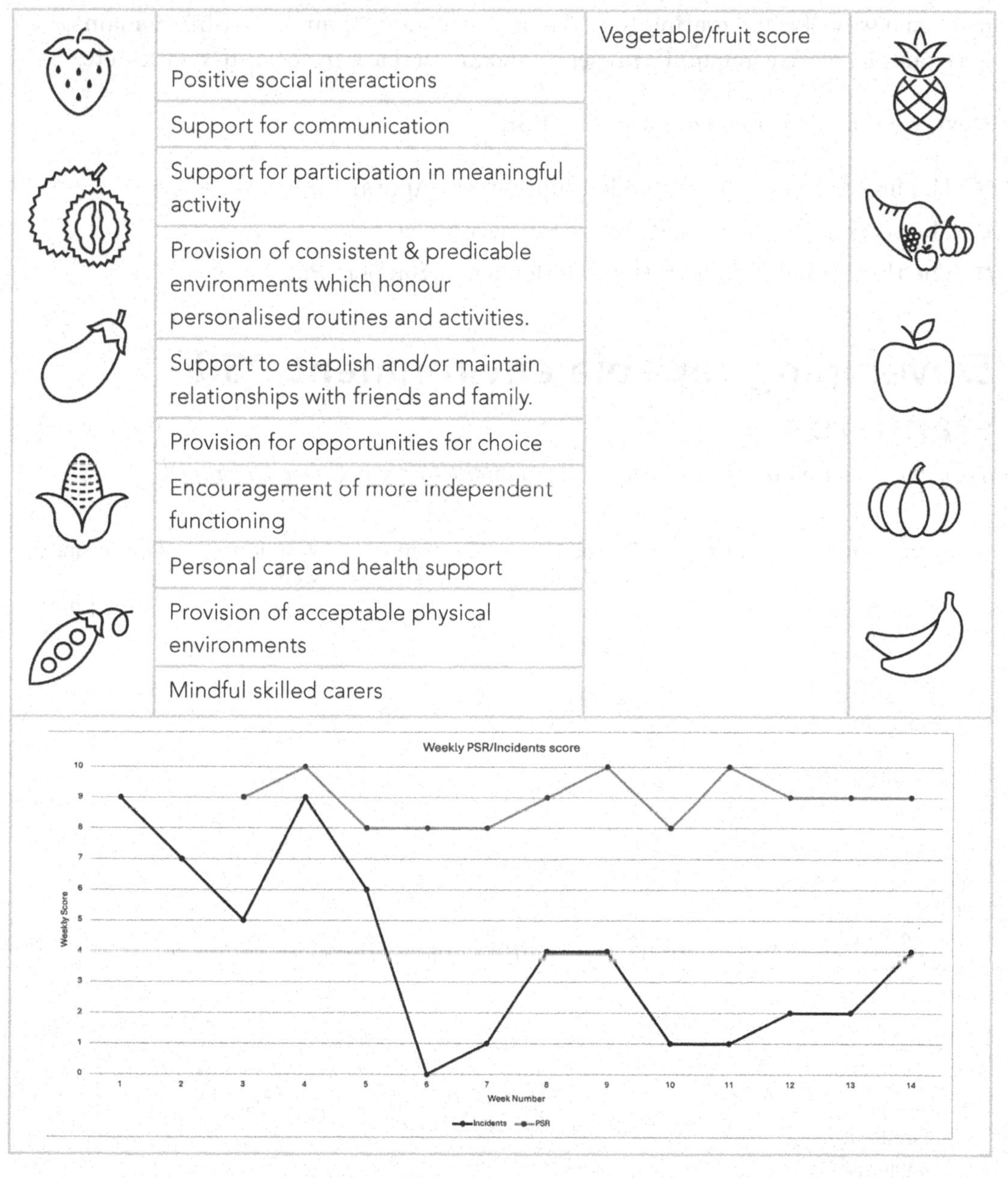

	Vegetable/fruit score
Positive social interactions	
Support for communication	
Support for participation in meaningful activity	
Provision of consistent & predicable environments which honour personalised routines and activities.	
Support to establish and/or maintain relationships with friends and family.	
Provision for opportunities for choice	
Encouragement of more independent functioning	
Personal care and health support	
Provision of acceptable physical environments	
Mindful skilled carers	

This image represents the weekly PSR score (ten a day), and it is mapped to the number of incidents of challenging behaviour for one individual. It can also be mapped to the scores for engagement and positive staff interactions (ASM Figure 7.4). This shows that where the PSR score increases there is typically a decrease in episodes of behaviours that challenge and improvements to the quality of support provided. This is just one way to use PSR data in terms of impact. It can also be used as a way of collaborating to make improvements to quality-of-life domains, for example, more community presence and an increase in social networks, etc.

Next, we provide three templates of a PSR.

- The first is linked to a Capable Environment Appraisal.
- The second is linked to the Active Support Measure.
- The third is based upon a Positive Behaviour Support Plan.

Developing capable environment PSR standards

This can be based on the Capable Environment Appraisal (see Chapter 2).

Characteristic	Standard	Process standard	Outcome standard	Working well	Opportunity for development
Positive social interactions					
Encouragement of more independent functioning					
Support to maintain/ establish relationships with friends and family					
Support for communication					
Support for participation in meaningful activities					

Enabling Capable Environments © Pavilion Publishing and Media Ltd and its licensors 2024.

Provision for opportunities for choice					
Mindful, skilled support workers					
Provision of acceptable physical environments					
Effective organisational contexts					
Effective management and support					
Provision of consistent predicable and personalised routines					

Developing a Person-Centred Active Support PSR

This can be based on the findings from the Active Support Measure (see Chapter 7).

Characteristic	Standard	Process standard	Outcome standard	Working well	Opportunity for development
Age appropriateness					
Real activities					
Choice of activities					
Demands presented carefully					

Task appropriately analysed					
Sufficient staff contact					
Graded assistance to ensure success					
Interpersonal warmth					
Staff notice and respond to client communication					
Staff work as a team					
Teaching is embedded in everyday activities					
Specific written plans are in routine use					

Enabling Capable Environments © Pavilion Publishing and Media Ltd and its licensors 2024.

PSR based upon a comprehensive Positive Behaviour Support Plan

Periodic Service Review

Petra Smyth

March 2023

PSR review date: ______________________________

Facilitator: ______________________________

Participants: ______________________________

	+/0
1. Periodic Service Review (PSR):	
a. Implementation: A '+' is scored if PSR graph shows at least two data points for previous 30 days.	
b. Progress: A '+' is scored if PSR graph shows a score of at least 85% or best score ever was achieved within previous 30 days.	
2. Data collection:	
a. Data Collection: A '+' is scored if ASM Sheet has been fully filled out for each day for the previous 7 days.	
b. Data Collection: A '+' is scored if Capable Environment Appraisal graph has been completed for this week.	
c. Summary Graphs: A '+' is scored if summary graphs of occurrence and episodic severity are up to date.	
d. Summary Graphs: A '+' is scored if summary graphs of meeting friends and family are up to date.	
3. Ecological strategies:	
Interpersonal environment:	
a. Staff protocol: Interaction style. A '+' is scored if there is a plan to direct staff supporting Petra in their communications and interactions with each other.	
b. Staff protocol: Separation. A '+' is scored if there is a protocol on file to direct staff supporting Petra in their communication with her friends and family.	
c. Communication Board. A '+' is scored if the communication board is on display and reflects the current days schedule.	
Programmatic environment:	
d. There is a plan and risk assessment completed for any new activity plus board maker symbol or photo to identify the activity.	

Enabling Capable Environments © Pavilion Publishing and Media Ltd and its licensors 2024.

Physical environment:	
e. A progress plan for redecoration has been devised with set target dates for completion.	
f. Storage areas and a chalk/drawing board have been established and are accessible.	
4. Positive programming:	
a. General skills.	
• Making a meal for family. A '+' is scored if the last scheduled family meal Petra cooked has been supported and the recipe steps were followed.	
• Calling friends and family. A '+' is scored if the last training session has been carried out and training data were collected and summarised.	
• Putting on karaoke machine. A '+' is scored if the last scheduled training session has been carried out and training data were collected and summarised.	
b. Functionally equivalent skills.	
• Requesting time with staff. A '+' is scored if the last scheduled training session has been carried out and training data were collected and summarised.	
c. Functionally related skills.	
• 'I don't understand'. A '+' is scored if the last scheduled training session has been carried out and training data were collected and summarised.	
d. Coping and tolerance skills.	
• Waiting in line. A '+' is scored if the last scheduled training session has been carried out and training data were collected and summarised.	
Focused support:	
a. Density of preferred activities. A '+' is scored if Petra's weekly diary shows that she has been to a community-based activity at least three times in the past week, taking part in a new community activity, i.e. one that has only been offered within the last month.	
5. Reactive strategies:	
a. Problem solving protocol. A '+' is scored if there are plans in the file indicating how staff are to respond to shouting behaviour, including the different levels of episodic severity that have been defined and the relevant responses to each.	
6. Staff development and management systems:	
a. Staff training. Records show that all staff, including seasonal are trained to the induction level of competence to work in a learning/ intellectual disability service. (Five identified courses.)	

Enabling Capable Environments © Pavilion Publishing and Media Ltd and its licensors 2024.

b. Support Plans. A '+' is scored if there is support plans to direct staff in how to support Petra in all aspects of her life and are in the agreed upon format. (Pro-rated credit is provided, e.g., 5/12=.42)	
c. Tiered training. A '+' is scored if staff training records indicate they have been trained to the third tier for each of Petra's support plans. (Pro-rated credit is provided.)	
d. Practice leadership coaching. A '+' is scored if a practice leader coaching session has been carried out for all support plans as scheduled for prior month and the agreed upon standard has been met. (Pro-rated credit is provided.)	
e. Team meetings.	
1. Protocol Sub-committee. A '+' is scored if last scheduled meeting was held and minutes show standard agenda was followed.	
2. Supervision. A '+' is scored if a supervision session was held in previous month for each staff member and minutes show standard agenda was followed.	
7. Quarterly review and progress report:	
a. A '+' is scored if last quarterly progress report follows standard format and is dated within prior four months	
Score achieved:	
Score possible:	
Percentage of score achieve to score possible:	

Discussion questions:

1. What will be the main driver for setting your PSR standards (Capable Environment Appraisal, Positive Behaviour Support Plan, or something else?)
2. What are the key components of PSR standards?
3. Think of the ways you can provide visual feedback from a PSR to your team.
4. When considering implementing a PSR, what roles do each team member need to consider in its development and implementation?

Enabling Capable Environments © Pavilion Publishing and Media Ltd and its licensors 2024.

Conclusion

- Where quality of support is lacking, the effects on people with intellectual disabilities can be harmful to them and their families.
- Quality of services and staff support is strongly associated with the quality-of-life outcomes for people with intellectual disabilities.
- Positive associations have been identified in several studies where improving the quality of interactions and practices has a positive association with quality of life and staff motivation.
- Staff who are supported in their application of daily practice and who are clear about their role report higher levels of job satisfaction.
- Implementation of a PSR has shown increased quality of staff support and engagement, a reduction in the need for external specialist support and improvements to the overall quality of services.
- Practice leadership is a critical element of implementing a PSR or any quality improvement system.
- The PSR is a 'living' document and, as such, is continuously updated and revised as agreed tasks, revised practices and responsibilities evolve.

 Enabling Capable Environments © Pavilion Publishing and Media Ltd and its licensors 2024.

Chapter 6: Practice leadership: Optimising a vision of practice

'The best practice leaders have taught me to opt for changing how things are done, not how things are spoken.' (Lovett, 1996)

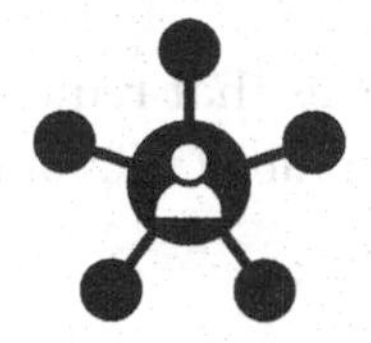

Chapter contents:

- What is practice leadership?
- Who are practice leaders?
- Motivating and training teams.
- Developing practices with a focus on quality of life.
- The 'practice' of leading.
- Barriers and enablers to supporting teams in person-centred approaches.

Learning outcomes

After reading this chapter and completing the suggested activities and reflection, the reader should be able to:

- Recognise the key components of the role of the practice leader.
- Identify how to support staff to implement a capable environment framework.
- Develop an understanding of how to review and evaluate engagement in meaningful activities.
- Understand the principles of coaching and mentoring in practice (including how to address barriers and promote resolutions to these).

Introduction

There has been a change in our understanding of what impacts the quality of life of individuals with intellectual disabilities. There was a belief, based on medical models of support, that resolving individual physical, emotional and behavioural factors would improve people's overall well-being, leading to improvements in their quality of life. However, due to increasing knowledge and a better understanding, this concept has evolved to recognise that quality of life increases through environmental changes, people's values, and how these contribute to well-being (personal, familial, community and societal) (Schalock, 2004). This understanding has led to considerable research and advances in practices to increase service delivery and the quality of life of individuals with an intellectual disability.

Common themes that arise in services that request specialist input relating to behaviours that challenge include some of the following:

- Support is poorly organised.
- There is limited personalised support; for example, staff may have attended communication training but lack the skills to implement this in their practice.
- A lack of training and support which focuses on engagement and participation.
- Organisational focus is predominantly on administrative duties, making managers less visible.
- Practice leaders are not readily available to support teams with implementing plans.

The Royal College of Psychiatrists (RCP) (2007) recommend that services should focus on improving a person's quality of life regardless of the level of intensity or frequency of behaviours that challenge. Furthermore, they identified that staff need training, support and clear guidance to promote positive interactions that increase participation, independence, choice and inclusion within local communities. In our experiences, there is often a focus on training but a lack of support for team members to implement these principles in practice. There is a tendency to provide training and then hope it translates into practice.

A train and hope it works model

Szabo *et al.* (2012) stress that training is rarely sufficient and there is a need for both workshops and on-the-job training. The combination of understanding what needs to happen and the evidence of why it needs to happen,

 Enabling Capable Environments © Pavilion Publishing and Media Ltd and its licensors 2024.

as well as the practical skills to make it happen, requires a more collaborative approach to ensure this works in practice. Practice leadership can help this process.

What is practice leadership?

Practice leadership is a fundamental factor that will have an impact on the quality of life of individuals. Managers are essential in developing and supporting frontline staff, building skills and influencing staff values (Bigby *et al.*, 2018).

In their work, Beadle-Brown *et al.* (2015) demonstrated that how well managers organise support has a direct influence on how well people with intellectual disabilities actively participate in their everyday lives. They found several skills that frontline managers might have that support good practice within learning/intellectual disability services. A number of these skills are focused on supporting service users directly, demonstrating good practice and supervising staff. Later, Bigby & Bould (2017) also showed that coaching, leading and supervising were critical in influencing staff practice. Beadle-Brown *et al.* (2015) agree, suggesting more is needed to be skilled at coaching. Managers must also be skilled at delivering the type of support they want to see. Sending staff on training programmes to increase quality-of-life measures or change practice is rarely sufficient; leaders must be able to provide on-the-job training.

Later studies by these authors show that a focus of practice leadership should be on quality-of-life outcomes for service users and that these are congruent with the principles of active support, which in turn will influence how staff act in practice.

Figure 6.1: Optimising change: a practice leadership model.

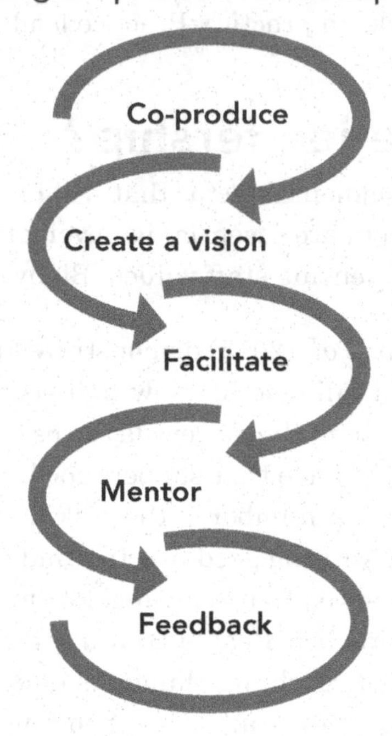

Figure 6.1, above, represents how we experience the role of a practice leader; this is someone who creates a co-produced vision of quality support and services. Practice leadership at its best helps to focus the role of staff to be more active and facilitative, more person-centred and enabling. However, for this to happen, there must be a shared vision of successful, meaningful support. Central to any support service, and to achieve this, staff must feel supported, guided and educated by those leading them and, crucially, those leaders must lead side by side, guiding and mentoring along the way. Practice leaders inspire us to be better at what we do and not just talk about change.

Who are practice leaders?

Practice leadership is the development and maintenance of a support team's skills and practice. This is achieved by people within the team adopting a leadership role. People in practice leadership roles focus on ensuring the attention of staff is on the quality of life of supported individuals, ensuring the right staff with the necessary skills are providing the right support to ensure people's needs and wishes are met. Practice leaders support this by modelling best practices, continuously appraising

 Enabling Capable Environments © Pavilion Publishing and Media Ltd and its licensors 2024.

staff practice, and ensuring staff teams are kept abreast with their progress concerning engagement, participation and relationship building (Bould *et al.*, 2016).

The person who takes on the role of practice leader may differ within different organisations due to job roles, titles, expectations, etc. However, the fundamental principles should always remain, namely: making it clear who within services holds this role, that the individual is aware of this, and has the skills and resources to perform the role effectively.

Hume *et al.* (2021) conducted a pilot study that focused on developing capable environments through practice leadership. Within their study, they spent considerable time working with the team to help them identify which role could facilitate this type of leadership. The best agents to make changes in this area were identified as the team leaders and senior support workers as they had the most influence in effecting change, given their role within services. This was because these individuals:

- Had positive relationships with the people being supported.
- Had close working relationships with the staff who worked directly with individuals being supported.
- Managed the day-to-day running of the service.
- They were based in the service/individual's homes.
- Provided supervision to staff teams.
- Conducted debriefings with staff after incidents or near misses.
- Oversaw the review of support with internal and external stakeholders.
- Developed and reviewed support plan documentation.

When deciding who should adopt the role of practice leader, a fundamental step is to clearly outline what this involves.

Practice leadership involves co-producing a shared vision of a successful service and supports

The practice leaders must:

- **Focus** on all aspects of service delivery, the individual's quality of life, and how the team supports this.

- **Allocate** and organise support to deliver on the shared vision when and how the individual wants/needs this.
- **Coach** and mentor good practice and provide feedback.
- **Review** the quality of support as outlined in the vision using a continuous improvement cycle.

Thinking space

Think about the school, service or environment you work in. Who would be the best person/people to take on the role of practice leader?
Consider:

- Who is best placed to keep a team focused on the quality of life of the people being supported?
- Who has the knowledge and skills to coach and mentor others to implement practice that is focused on quality of life?
- Who knows the person and those who deliver direct support well?
- Who can observe and provide feedback?

A shared vision means practice leaders have something to lead on

Co-production in the context of practice leadership is a shift in thinking about the cultural structures and practices of teams, it sharpens our focus on people having an equal role in the design and delivery of services.

Thinking space

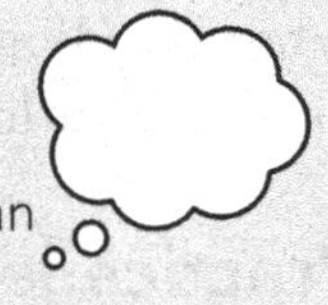

Research, such as Beadle-Brown *et al.* (2015) shows that this type of practice leadership is generally not present in services for people with an intellectual disability.

Consider a service you have worked in:

- Think about an occasion in which coaching and mentoring were not provided.
- Now think of services in which this did occur.
- What did this look like?
- What influence did this have on you or the colleagues you worked with?

 Enabling Capable Environments © Pavilion Publishing and Media Ltd and its licensors 2024.

If we consider some of the questions that are relevant to 'staff performance', they might include:

- Do staff have the knowledge to know what to do?
- Do they have the skills to do what is needed, when it's needed?
- Are they motivated to do this?
- Is feedback provided from multiple sources including direct feedback in practice?

A practice leader is critical in bridging the gaps that occur in this cycle (Figure 6.2).

Figure 6.2: Supporting staff practice

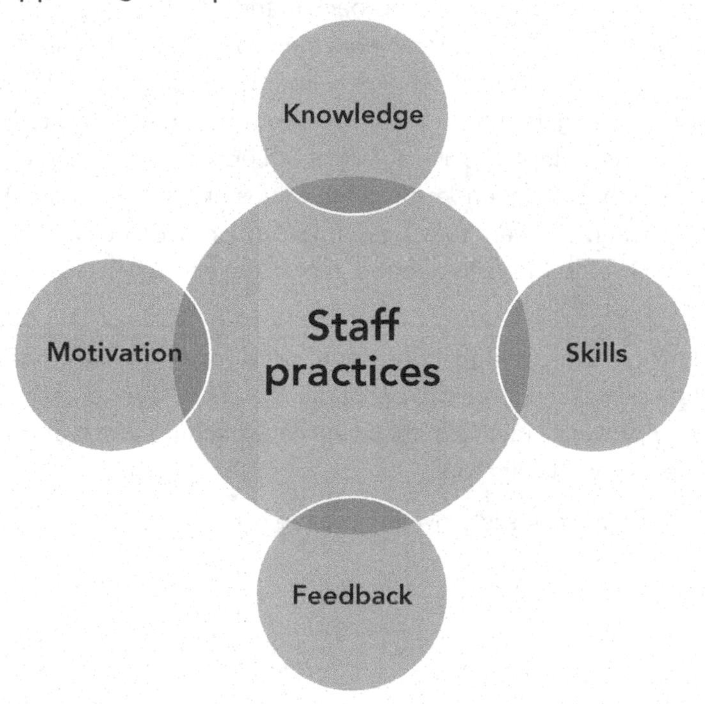

Training approaches

Beadle-Brown *et al.* (2015) state that how adults with intellectual disabilities can participate in everyday life depends on how support is organised by leaders. In addition, and as already discussed, they report that there are several leadership skills that support good practice within services. A number of these skills focus on supporting people with an intellectual disability themselves, demonstrating good practice to others, as well as supervising and mentoring staff in their good practice.

Enabling Capable Environments © Pavilion Publishing and Media Ltd and its licensors 2024.

It is not enough for a practice leader to be skilled at coaching, they must also be skilled at the type of support they want to see. Bigby & Bould (2017) identify that practice leaders who are skilled at providing support are better placed to then provide coaching, and be able to lead and supervise others, and these are crucial in influencing staff practice.

Case study: knowledge and skills

Research shows that 'whole environment training [is needed] to improve the quality of support by staff teams in supported accommodation settings' (Mansell *et al.*,1994). Inspired by this, Hume *et al.* (2021) adopted this approach in their pilot programme using the capable environments framework (see Chapter 2: Enabling capable environments) to design a whole environment training which included a combination of coaching, mentoring and classroom-based learning to best meet the needs of services. Adopting such an approach ensures that people have the knowledge about what to do, understand the values of why it needs to be done, and maintain the motivation to want to achieve it. With opportunities for coaching and mentoring, they develop the skills needed in practice and receive feedback on their performance of these skills.

In this pilot, a programme of eight classroom-based training workshops was developed. Between each workshop, participants worked through specific activities that related to improving practice in their service. Coaching and mentoring were provided by the training facilitators.

A summary of these activities is provided in table 6.1.

 Enabling Capable Environments © Pavilion Publishing and Media Ltd and its licensors 2024.

Table 6.1: Hume *et al.* (2021) training programme				
Session	**Content**	**Participant activity**	**Training facilitator activity**	**Output**
1	Values-based support (Lovett, 1996; Sailor *et al*, 2010) Capable environment framework adapted to include evidence for current support and opportunities for development (McGill *et al*, 2014; 2020)	Review support to a focal person and complete appraisal tool (see Chapter 2: Enabling capable environments)	Guide appraisal of current support	Individual support plan developed using characteristics of the capable environment.
2	Overview of positive behaviour support (Gore *et al.*, 2013); person-centred active support (PCAS) (Beadle-Brown *et al*, 2012).	Identify key areas of active support for focal person using the four principles of PCAS.	Guide development of detailed plans that incorporate characteristics of capable environment framework	Detailed plan for providing PCAS
3	Periodic Service Review (PSR) of the plan (LaVigna *et al.*, 1994)	Define performance standards and create individual PSR specifying: WHAT staff should do in OBSERVABLE terms; WHEN they should do it; WHO is responsible for each action; HOW everyone will know the action has been carried out (see Chapter 5: Periodic Service Review)	Guide development of PSR	PSR was created with a visual graph to allow for monitoring

4	Using practice leadership to embed active support and capable environments. (Beadle-Brown *et al*, 2015)	Training and mentoring other staff using a practice leadership approach	Guide development of plans to prevent challenging behaviour.	Provision of daily x 15 minutes feedback to team members
5	Identify barriers and enablers to the implementation process (Mansell *et al*, 2008)	Develop a plan to promote the implementation	Coach implementation skills such as leading team meetings, prioritising tasks, and addressing concerns in practice	Implementation skills practised
6	Resolution Strategies (Spicer & Crates, 2016)	Create resolution (reactive) strategies for the focal person.	Guide development of plans for successful resolution of incidents of challenging behaviour	Resolution strategies developed
7	Assessing and understanding the meaning of behaviour (O'Neil *et al*, 2015)	Define the focal person's behaviours that challenge and assess their functions	Guide to analyse data and produce a formulation	Person-centred understanding of the focal person's behaviour
8	Enabling opportunities and developing skills (Beadle-Brown *et al*, 2012)	Identify opportunities for engagement; develop functional (fun) skills	Facilitate the development of plan and provide direct mentoring in service to implement and coach practice leadership	Plan to develop a skill that is functionally equivalent to challenging behaviour

In this pilot programme, the training facilitators initially undertook the core activities of the practice leader as a means of coaching the participants into their role as future practice leads.

Enabling Capable Environments © Pavilion Publishing and Media Ltd and its licensors 2024.

Figure 6.3: Scaffolding practice leadership (five tiers to competency)

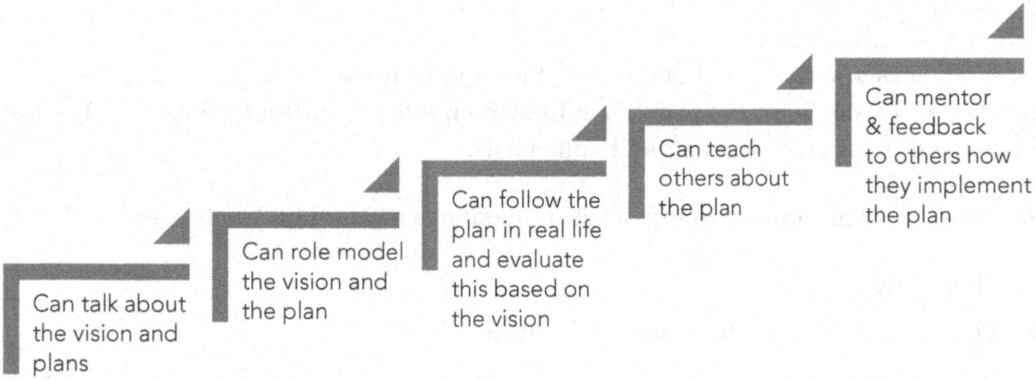

The participants of this pilot training (Hume *et al.*, 2021) were assisted in developing support plans and a quality improvement process to support this, i.e. Periodic Service Review (PSR) (see Chapter 5) based on the capable environment's framework (see Chapter 2). These were designed around their focus person as part of the 'classroom-based training'. A critical element of the programme involved the use of a scaffolding method of coaching and mentoring (Figure 6.3) that was provided in both group and one-to-one sessions as well as in practice. This involved coaching on spending time with staff, giving feedback and modelling good practice.

The participants were then able to engage with the training facilitators and use this as an opportunity to reflect on success and opportunities for further development of their role as practice leaders. A key part of this engagement was to support developing practice leads to 'practise' how to review the quality of the support provided and how to maximise opportunities to feed this back to staff at supervision, in practice (in vivo) or at team meetings. The main aim was to achieve a change in how the group viewed their role as practice leaders within the service and the impact they can have on motivating and engaging staff teams in their role as ambassadors for creating capable environments.

Motivation

Providing information or knowledge is an important factor in enhancing the motivation of staff teams. However, there can be other factors which can impede this. Most organisations will have statements in their organisation mission statements, job descriptions and job advertisements that refer to 'having good values' or encourage people to apply for posts if they have good values (this can be followed by a statement that 'experience not essential as full training will be provided…').

Nevertheless, the concept of personal values and that what you do is valued is rarely addressed as part of people's induction or, indeed, within feedback (if they get any) about what they do on a day-to-day basis.

Two key areas are known to impact staff member's motivation levels are:

- Their values.
- Their perceptions of the managers' values

Staff values

When speaking about values, it is understood that everyone holds their own, which may or may not be in opposition to the type of values that they need when providing support as part of their job role. The focus for a practice leader is to understand what support staff require to reconcile personal and professional values so that they can provide good person-centred support. This can be done through supervision, providing staff with additional support such as a mentor, training, having a focus on person-centred support at team meetings, etc.

Perceptions of managers' values

How staff perceive what managers value also contributes to their motivation. If staff experience the contribution or presence of managers in a service as negative, they are more likely to engage in activities which avoid this negativity.

Some examples of this include:

- Staff feel that managers are only interested in incident forms or checklists. As a result, they may prioritise or only focus on these tasks, possibly resulting in less time spent on other tasks, such as encouraging engagement and participation.
- If there is a perception that a manager expects staff to know how to support in all areas at all times based on written instructions or because that member of staff has attended training, staff feeling uncertain or anxious about key activities may avoid them. They may make excuses for why they are not done, suggesting they are too risky, rather than seeking guidance and support.
- Staff may feel that managers don't understand that they are finding parts of their job difficult and feel they are left to get on with it. Such situations can

 Enabling Capable Environments © Pavilion Publishing and Media Ltd and its licensors 2024.

lead staff to form narratives that managers don't know anything about how to provide support and, therefore, they do not seek their support and may choose to provide what they think is best. If the person is using supports that do not meet the individual's needs or is unable to lead the whole team, this could have negative consequences.

For practice leaders, they must understand their role in preventing such cultures from developing in their services. Practice leaders must ensure that teams feel valued in what they do, that success is celebrated, and that the opportunity to develop and improve their practice in the context of people having a good life becomes the narrative and culture of the service.

Using feedback to develop practice: a focus on quality of life

As mentioned in Chapter 2, practice leaders can use the findings from their capable environments appraisal to lead a team in developing the quality of the support provided within their services. There is strong evidence that when a person has their needs met (i.e. communication, health, a suitable home, sensory needs, relationships, and positive interactions with others, as well as predictable routines and activities), they are much more likely to enjoy a higher quality of life and less likely to present with behaviours that are perceived or labelled as challenging.

While many services understand that a good quality of life is core to human rights, this does not always translate to a priority focus in practice. To achieve this, leaders must have conversations with those supporting the person that are based on the quality of life of the individuals they support, asking questions that focus on what each member of staff has done to impact someone's quality of life. Quality of life outcomes should be the first agenda item of all formal meetings, as well as the first questions asked in impromptu conversations. The capable environments framework is one way for services and teams to think about the key areas which will improve the quality of life of the people they support.

Enabling Capable Environments © Pavilion Publishing and Media Ltd and its licensors 2024.

Figure 6.4: The 'practice' of leading

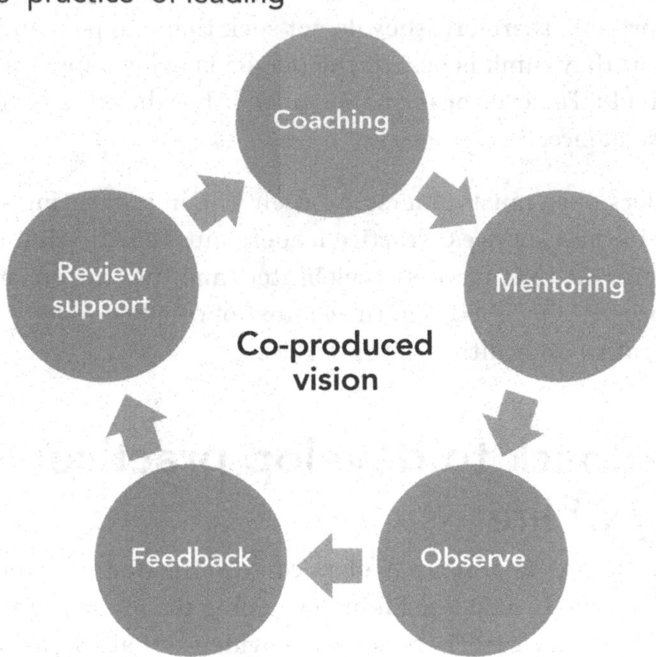

Figure 6.4 shows the five characteristics that are essential in providing practice leadership and maintaining a co-produced vision of support.

Coaching and mentoring

Practice leaders spend time building relationships with staff members and the people they support, ensuring they know them well. With this knowledge, they can model and facilitate good support approaches. Visiting a service once every few weeks or months is not sufficient to truly know and understand both the staff team and the people receiving support. While external professionals may need to work in this way due to their job role and may provide some of the more technical understanding around behaviours that challenge, the role of the practice leader is different. They need to be able to work with people to fully understand what type of support is needed and the approaches required to embed this into day-to-day practice. To do this, the practice leader needs to appreciate what support the team need, this can involve bringing ideas together and trying out approaches to see how and why they work or, indeed, if some approaches don't work. Once appropriate support strategies are identified, agreed upon and established, it is the role of the practice leader to work with the team to model these strategies.

 Enabling Capable Environments © Pavilion Publishing and Media Ltd and its licensors 2024.

An example of this is found in the pilot study by Hume *et al.* (2021). Coaching and mentoring were provided by the trainers to the trainee practice leaders. This involved developing the participant's skills in observation and feedback. This was achieved by:

- Clearly explaining the processes involved in observation and feedback.
- Providing written information that supported the ability to conduct observations and provide feedback.
- Allowing time for questions, comments and problem-solving until trainees felt confident.
- Offering role-play and practice scenarios alongside feedback.
- Conducting observations of trainee practice leaders as they implement their skills in practice.
- Providing prompts and support during observations.
- Based on observations, providing written and verbal feedback to trainees.

The fundamental components of coaching and mentoring were not limited to the trainee practice leader but were implemented throughout the programme at all levels. As well as teaching trainees how to provide coaching and mentoring to their staff, trainers were concurrently providing coaching and mentoring to the trainees, modelling good practice.

Trainee practice leaders were supported in their practice area through coaching and mentoring provided by trainers, and in turn, they then supported staff teams through in-person coaching and mentoring.

Direct observations

Once staff are trained in the agreed support, practice leaders should remain a consistent source of support, both remotely and in practice with direct mentoring. Without this, it is easy for teams to become stuck and minor practice issues can quickly become obstacles. Coaching and observations should include how all elements of support are being put into practice, and they should be done in a structured and systematic way. This means that any observation should be related directly to the PBS (Positive Behaviour Support) plan, the capable environment appraisal or other person-centred framework.

One way of ensuring this is to design an observation guide (Appendix 3: Guide for Observation) for the specific area of support that you are observing. (i.e., the

Enabling Capable Environments © Pavilion Publishing and Media Ltd and its licensors 2024.

consistent use of a particular communication system). Practice leaders need to ensure that they are available at various times to support direct observations across the weekly staff schedule so that they gain a representative understanding of how the team works and identify areas of good practice and opportunities for development. Feedback, however, should be done on an individual basis.

Case study

In Hume *et al.*'s (2021) pilot programme, the trainee practice leaders were supported to create a PSR based on the capable environment framework. Once a PSR standard had been created for each component of the framework, the trainee practice leader was able to organise direct observations in a structured and systematic way. This allowed them to plan their observations around the rest of their workload on any given shift.

The example below shows how a PSR standard was agreed upon for Jonah.

Jonah's person-centred plan shows he would like to attend a drama class, go to the theatre and visit places with Monet paintings or pictures.

What	Jonah's weekly planner includes at least two opportunities, chosen by him, for a culture community-based activity.
When	Each Sunday morning when Johan is planning his week ahead.
Who	Practice lead to directly observe support staff following 'choosing activities' support plan.
How	Direct observation of weekly planner being created. Records state that activities occurred (unless cancelled by venue). Artefact from attending the event

In this example, there is a clearly defined time that the practice leader can carry out this observation (on a Sunday morning). This allows the observation to be planned. It is important to ensure that observations take place. Often observations are missed or forgotten about due to not being planned or not having a clearly defined process. In addition, being available and present, directly observing, facilitates the opportunity for discussion or any coaching that may be needed in practice.

 Enabling Capable Environments © Pavilion Publishing and Media Ltd and its licensors 2024.

Providing feedback

Practice leaders need to tell staff what worked well and why, and agree on future opportunities for development with them, where needed. Whether it is maximising participation and engagement or following a specific support plan, practice leaders need to be able to engage with staff about what works well. Often, we focus too much on pointing out errors, but by focusing on what worked well, we can build on skills and motivation. Practice leaders providing feedback about practices they see supports the team and helps to recognise that what they do is essential and valued. Opportunities to observe and coach staff in practice should occur at regular planned intervals, but impromptu presence at the service ensures that leaders are visible and can help understand the needs of the team. Building this into regular practice helps staff understand the role of the practice leader and that this is a normal part of what happens at work.

Case study

A key factor in providing feedback is to ensure that this is a positive experience. Historically, staff have often associated managers' presence or feedback as something negative and this risks teams concealing the problems they face. Previous negative experiences of feedback can lead staff members to view any feedback they receive as critical of their practice. It is important to think about the type of language used, especially if the feedback may include addressing concerns identified during observations. In Hume *et al.*'s (2021) pilot programme, they were mindful to use language that allowed practice leaders to discuss issues in a positive and solution focused way. If a practice leader had carried out an observation and was required to give feedback to staff about areas of their practice, they summarised this under the heading 'opportunities for development'. The idea is to remove the perception from frontline staff that all feedback is critical of them. In the pilot programme, they ensured that the practice leader had a role to play in these 'opportunities for development', reinforcing the process as collaborative and supportive.

Reviewing support

A continuous review of the support being provided is the best way to ensure we are always supporting people as best as we can. Again, such ongoing review is not always a consistent focus of services. Often, services will focus intensely on a particular support or project for a short period and ensure resources are available to implement this. This is frequently seen when services are expecting a formal (external) inspection or review from a regulatory body.

What most services fail to do is review this support in a systematic, dynamic way. This leads to common service issues such as:

- Staff support is inconsistent.
- New staff have no knowledge of existing plans.
- Staff develop their own practices.
- Staff become demoralised if they see no positive changes.

As discussed in the PSR chapter, the pilot programme used a PSR as the critical tool in evaluating the implementation of the capable environment's framework. However, regardless of how well a PSR or any tool for reviewing support is, it is only useful if it is co-produced, co-evaluated and used consistently. This is where practice leadership is vital. Practice leaders must ensure that they create a system where this review can take place with input from all staff involved. Through the pilot programme, Hume *et al.* (2021) worked with frontline managers to identify opportunities for this to happen. Some examples of these are detailed as follows:

Supervision with staff:

- Focus on the quality of life of the people they are supporting.
- Discuss and review how staff are doing this and if there are any concerns or whether further support is needed.
- Provide feedback from direct observation as well as listen to staff views. Agree on any changes that may be required.
- Provide guidance and mentoring to improve what they do.

Team meetings:

- Review how well the team is enabling people to engage in meaningful activity and relationships.
- Review the balance of activities, consistency of approach and pursuit of goals of inclusion, independence and choice.
- Review weekly PSR scores.
- Identify successes and celebrate them.

 Enabling Capable Environments © Pavilion Publishing and Media Ltd and its licensors 2024.

- Ensure safe supportive environments in which concerns or difficulties can be raised.
- Identify any changes that may need to be made and agree on who is responsible and when they will be completed.

Multi-disciplinary meetings:

- Involve other professionals who are involved in the support (PBS team, speech and language, occupational therapy) to allow for changes to support and further input etc.

Thinking space

When you arrive to observe a staff member providing support you find them sitting down reading a newspaper while the person they are supporting is sitting on the chair staring into space. Looking at the activity timetable, the person was meant to be supported to go to the shops. The staff member asked them if they needed anything from the shop and they said they did not, so they stayed at home.

In your role as a practice leader, what might you do both during and after the observation?

In the above scenario, it is important to ensure the person supported gets the engagement and interaction needed. As a practice leader, you will need to consider how you address this. You can do this by:

1. Saying hello to the supported person and asking if there is something they would like to do. If possible, ask another member of staff who knows the person well to support the individual to engage in that task while you speak to the original member of staff.
2. Approaching the member of staff openly and non-confrontationally, ask them if they know how to support the person to participate in their shopping trip and/or ways to support meaningful engagement and participation if the person chooses not to go shopping.
3. Reviewing the support plan documents together. Discuss each step and ensure the staff member has time to ask questions.
4. Role-playing the plan to enhance the member of staff's skills.

5. Ensuring the member of staff feels confident in the steps of the plan.
6. Supporting the staff member to implement their learning in practice. Remain with the staff member as they do this, offering feedback and support to implement the support plan.
7. Praising the staff member. Be specific and clear about what they are doing well and what changes may need to be made.
8. Later, when this does not interrupt the supported person's chosen routines/activities, review the implementation of the plan with the staff member.

Barriers and enablers to supporting staff practice

Barriers for managers

Frontline managers are expected to function in both a managerial and leadership capacity. The reality within services, however, is that they usually prioritise their management and administrative tasks over the leadership responsibilities of their role. This is usually due to organisational urgencies and regulatory requirements being seen as the priority, and this is primarily what managers are monitored and assessed on. It would not be uncommon within services to have a frontline manager spend most of their time in an office as opposed to being in the service, supporting staff as a practice leader.

If frontline managers are expected to be practice leaders, then it is vital to identify and resolve barriers that may impact their ability to do so. It is important to note that frontline managers may not always be best placed to adopt the role of practice leader due to other competing responsibilities. Here, it is completely appropriate and indeed necessary that someone else in the team is supported to undertake this role.

Barriers for support staff

A similar comment can be applied to direct support staff. A support worker's ability to provide good support is predicted by several factors:

- Motivation.
- Values.
- Monitoring.

Enabling Capable Environments © Pavilion Publishing and Media Ltd and its licensors 2024.

- Skill level of team members.
- Organisational issues such as a shortage of staff and rotas.
- Lack of routines and consistency.
- Skill issues such as a lack of staff training – staff may not have had sufficient training to ensure they understand the importance of active participation and ways in which they can support it.
- Lack of time – time restraints are a particularly common barrier that can lead to an increased temptation for a support worker to take over tasks for a service – doing for the person rather than with the person.

Case example

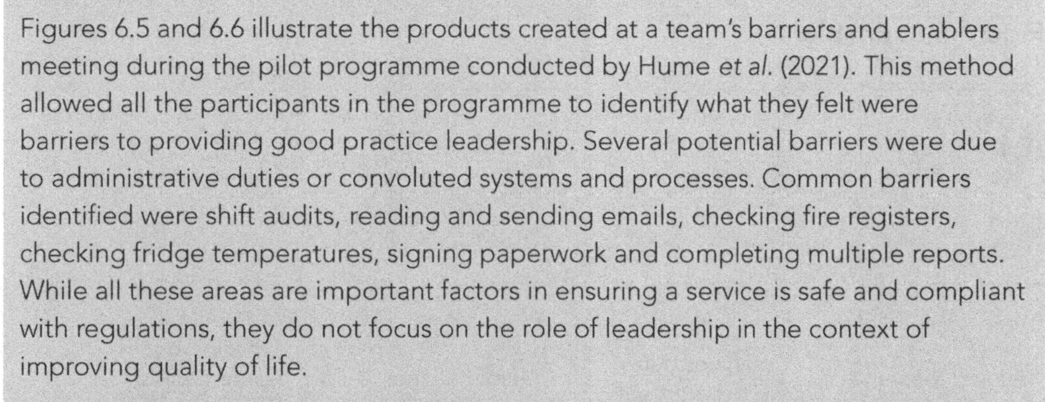

It was essential within the development of the Hume *et al.* (2021) pilot programme that key barrier-resolution skills were developed. We know situations within services are ever-changing and barriers can prevent good support from happening. It was crucial to teach practice leaders to identify barriers quickly and resolve them. Key skills such as leading team meetings, listening and addressing concerns, changing plans if there was no contextual fit, and showing the skills in practice were developed.

Figures 6.5 and 6.6 illustrate the products created at a team's barriers and enablers meeting during the pilot programme conducted by Hume *et al.* (2021). This method allowed all the participants in the programme to identify what they felt were barriers to providing good practice leadership. Several potential barriers were due to administrative duties or convoluted systems and processes. Common barriers identified were shift audits, reading and sending emails, checking fire registers, checking fridge temperatures, signing paperwork and completing multiple reports. While all these areas are important factors in ensuring a service is safe and compliant with regulations, they do not focus on the role of leadership in the context of improving quality of life.

Once these barriers had been identified, the group then listed key enablers. This then allowed them to identify and address common themes. As part of the process, once enablers or potential resolutions were identified, for the most part, the team themselves were able to implement the solutions. Those they could not resolve themselves were referred to more senior members of the team structure. Allowing teams to identify barriers and enablers to providing good support is one of the ways co-production empowers services to be more dynamic and solution-focused in their approaches.

Enabling Capable Environments © Pavilion Publishing and Media Ltd and its licensors 2024.

Figure 6.5: Barriers

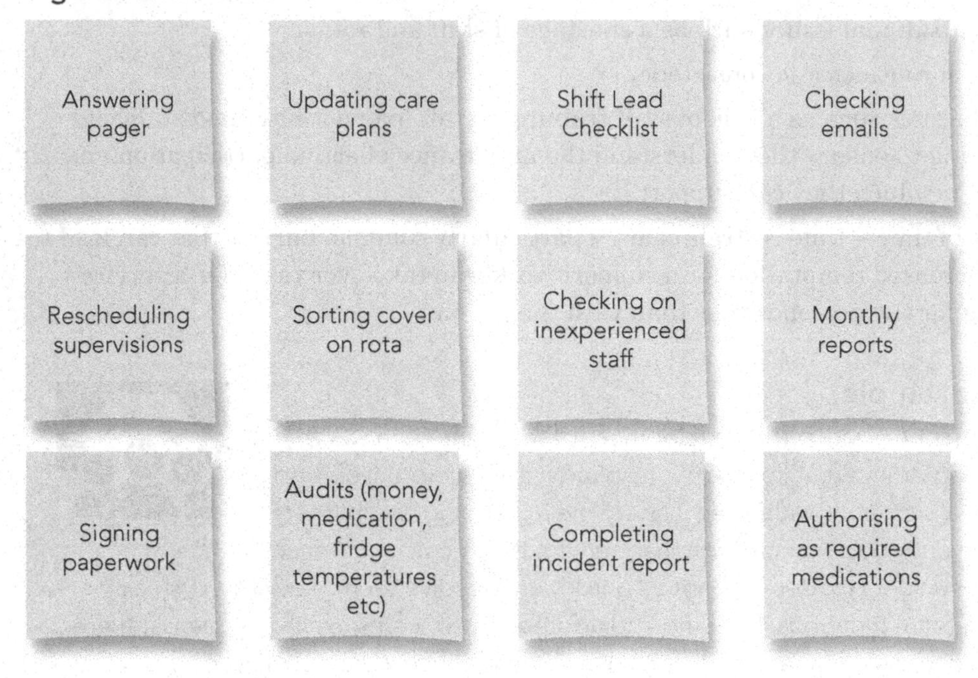

Figure 6.6: Enablers

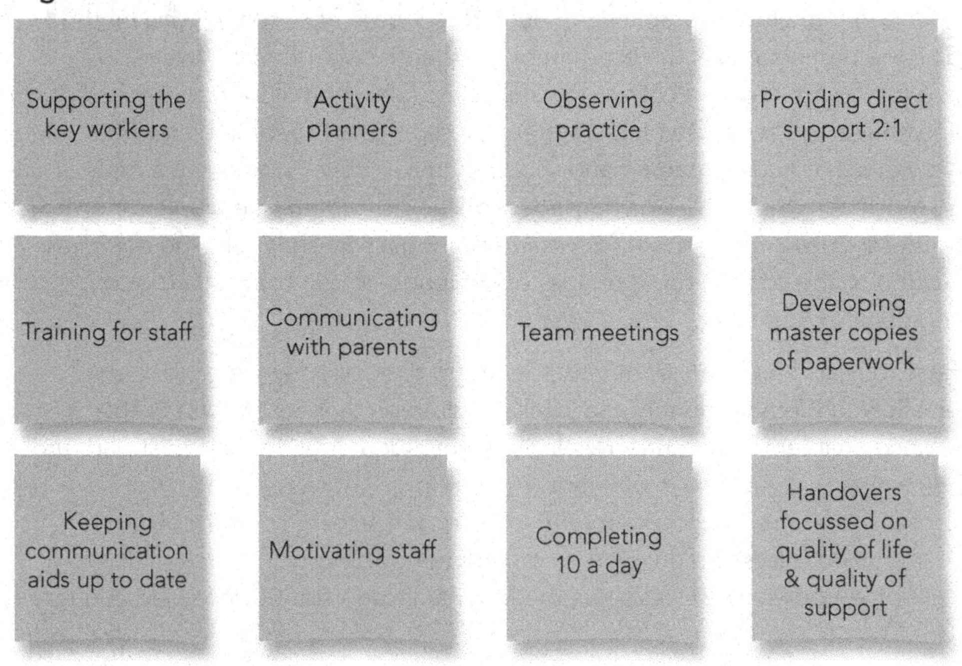

 Enabling Capable Environments © Pavilion Publishing and Media Ltd and its licensors 2024.

Thinking space

Although frontline staff have a key role in implementing person-centred support, they cannot do this without the support of managers and supervisors. Think about what you need to change to enable staff to provide person-centred active support.

You may find it helpful to think about the following headings (adapted from Beadle-Brown, Murphy & Bradshaw, 2017)):

1. How are you going to provide practice leadership? Consider coaching/modelling

- Plan time to observe practice, offer prompts and suggestions for changing practice, and provide feedback on how well supports were implemented.
- Ensure you are present and visible in your classroom and services, to allow staff teams to ask questions.

Giving feedback

- Make sure feedback is specific to what has been observed. Do not discuss anything that was not part of the observation or things that you may have heard that have happened – you would raise these at a different time.
- Think about where you would provide feedback so no one else can hear, the person feels able to concentrate on your feedback, and to ask questions, etc.

Reviewing support

- Plan time to review support plans and notes on how they are implemented (i.e. handover, running notes, communication book, etc.)
- You may also need to consider reviewing the highest priority plans initially or only doing a certain number at any one time etc.

2. How are you going to put active support/capable environments on the supervision agenda so that staff performance can be reviewed and improved?

- Develop a set agenda for the beginning or end of all supervision sessions.
- Ensure observations are equally shared across the staff team, across a specified period. You want to be able to observe all staff.
- Plan time for observations and for providing feedback.

3. Is there anything that needs to be changed in the environment or the resources available and what should you do about that? Consider capable environments appraisal.

4. How are you going to motivate staff to provide person-centred support? Consider:

Rotas/staff timetables

- Plan enough time for staff to implement plans effectively.
- Ensure all staff have scheduled time to observe new plans being implemented by others.

Values

- Ensure this is a set agenda point in team meetings, supervisions and training.

Skill level

- Ensure learning is delivered in different ways (i.e., written documentation, observing others, role-play and feedback).

Incentives

- Plan friendly ways that focus on how well plans are being implemented.
- Praise staff who do well at team meetings or through communication boards.

5. How are you going manage situations in which staff are nervous or reluctant to make changes to practice? Consider some of the following:

Supervision

- Plan time to discuss this fully.
- Review plans together, and allow time to ask questions or raise concerns.
- Make changes to plans if others identify factors that may impede its implementation.

Debrief

- Plan time to review practice.

Performance management

- Set clear achievable goals.
- Review these together.

Staffing support

- Review the scaffolding of support plans model in Chapter 3.

6. What staff development issues do you need to consider?

In doing this, you should also identify what support you need to achieve these things and be prepared to raise this in your supervision with your own manager.

 Enabling Capable Environments © Pavilion Publishing and Media Ltd and its licensors 2024.

Conclusion

- Practice leaders must support teams by coaching, modelling and mentoring.
- Understanding what motivates the staff team is crucial.
- Staff providing direct support must see the benefits of practice leadership to their role and feel included and supported.
- Whole-environment training is vital.
- Barriers to providing good support should be openly identified and discussed, but the key is to facilitate a process that identifies the enablers of good support.
- Review, review, review.

Enabling Capable Environments © Pavilion Publishing and Media Ltd and its licensors 2024.

Chapter 7: Person-Centred Active Support

'People's lives are usually enhanced when they benefit from a variety of activities each day; an active network of friends, neighbours, relatives and acquaintances, reflecting the personal preferences of the individual.' (Carr *et al.*, 1994, p112)

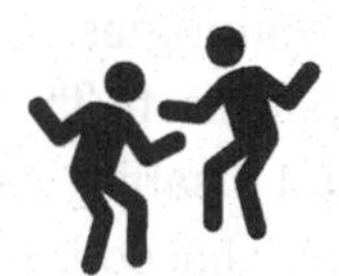

Chapter contents:

- What is meant by Person-Centred Active Support (PCAS) and why it is important?
- The importance of meaningful engagement.
- The four principles of PCAS.
- Enhancing opportunities for PCAS and overcoming barriers related to implementation.
- Developing plans and implementing PCAS practices.
- Paving the way to success.

Learning outcomes

After reading this chapter and completing the suggested activities and reflection, the reader should be able to:

- Identify the components of Person-Centred Active Support.
- Understand how Person-Centred Active Support can enhance the quality of support and people's quality of life.
- Apply the principles of Person-Centred Active Support to the development of support planning and their practice.

- Understand implementation approaches such as The Scaffolding Approach: moving from knowing to doing.

What is Person-Centred Active Support?

Person-Centred Active Support (PCAS) is an approach to supporting individuals, irrespective of disability or need, to participate in meaningful activities and relationships. This approach was developed from work by Mansell *et al.* (1983; 1987). They identified that people with an intellectual disability in institutionalised settings did not spend time engaged in any meaningful activity, were instead inactive or spent time engaged in 'meaningless' activities, and were likely to have limited engagement with their support staff. This was especially the case for people with severe and profound intellectual disabilities. Originally based on the support provided at one of the first community-based homes (Mansell *et al.*, 1983; 1987), Person-Centred Active Support has gathered momentum across the UK and is now widely used in supported living settings (McKim, 2021).

Since its development, PCAS continues to be used widely and has gathered a large evidence base (Mansell & Beadle-Brown., 2012; Bigby & Beadle-Brown., 2016). Evidence suggests that PCAS can increase: engagement (Baker *et al.*, 2017), independence, choice (Mansell & Beadle-Brown., 2012), community activities, social activities, interactions and understanding between supported individuals and their staff (Baker *et al.*, 2017) and can reduce behaviours that challenge (Mansell & Beadle-Brown, 2012).

Why is PCAS important?

When services are not organised, services and staff teams may lack focus and vision. This can lead to services becoming more focused on the completion of tasks, rather than focusing on including people with intellectual disabilities in all aspects of their lives and support. The consequence of this is staff members *doing* for rather than *with* and feeling compelled to complete daily (mundane) tasks in a mistaken belief that this indicates they are doing their jobs well. This type of approach may even be supported by managers or, be a result of staff not knowing what they should be doing so instead they complete tasks they are more confident in achieving, for example, if people are observed cleaning, cooking, filling in paperwork, and remaining busy (even if the person being supported is not involved), they likely won't be criticised. Unfortunately, this scenario results in higher levels of disengagement, disempowerment and dependency for people receiving support.

 Enabling Capable Environments © Pavilion Publishing and Media Ltd and its licensors 2024.

This has been likened to a 'hotel model' of support; a term used by Mansell (2007) to illustrate an institutional style setting, organised around staff and service needs rather than the needs of those being supported.

Figure 7.1: Hotel Model: Circle of Disempowerment (adapted from Mansell, 2007)

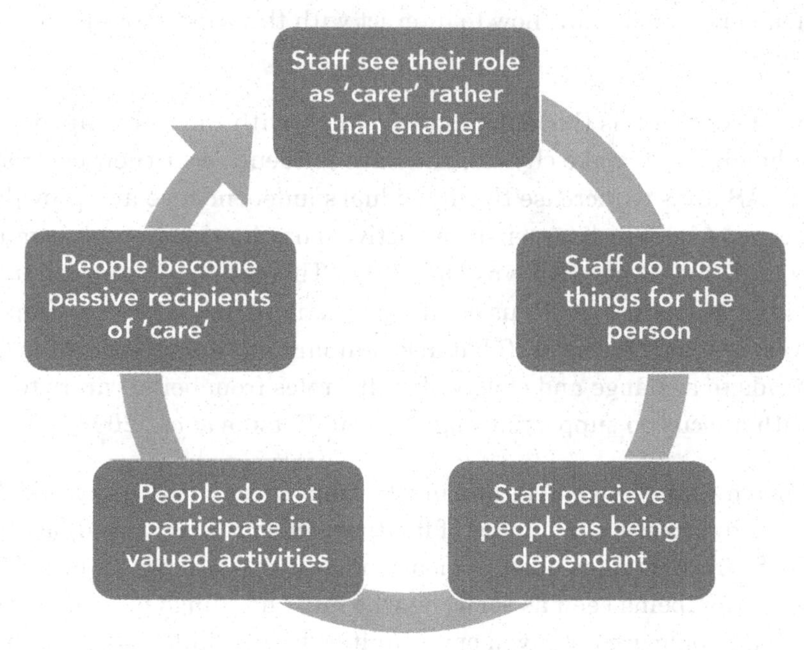

Figure 6.1 shows a representation of what Mansell (2007) viewed as the 'hotel model' of support. In this model, staff perceive the individual with an intellectual disability as being dependent on them and their support and feel they are responsible for doing things for them. They see their role as a 'carer role ' or someone who does things for a person, rather than as an 'enabler'. This results in staff doing most things for the person rather than creating opportunities for the person to participate, with limited time spent interacting with or assisting the person being supported. Staff members may also feel apprehensive about trying new things or be unaware of how to support the person to be involved, leading to an inability to develop goals or activities that the person being supported could do. The consequence is that the person does not participate in valued activities and spends most of their time doing very little (Mansell, 2007). The 'hotel model' has several negative outcomes:

- People do not get to use the skills they have and may forget how to do things they previously could do.

- The opportunity to experience and learn new skills does not happen.
- The person will not be encouraged and supported to participate in activities that directly relate to their own lives.
- The person may lose motivation and confidence and behaviour that we find challenging is more likely to occur.
- Staff members do not know how to interact with the person or support them in a way they need.

A key principle of PCAS is the belief that everyone, with the right support, can contribute, be involved, make choices, and have influence over their environment and lives. PCAS aims to increase the individual's independence and provide them with more control in their lives, ensuring active participation in their community (Mansell *et al.*, 2004, Beadle-Brown *et al.*, 2017). This is achieved by ensuring supported individuals are the focus of all tasks/activities that have an impact on their lives, not just the big stuff but also ordinary day-to-day activities. This approach leads to a change and clarity of staff's roles from being carers to being enablers with a focus on supporting engagement (Totsika *et al.*, 2008).

It is well known that engagement and involvement in activities, particularly those you like, leads to increases in quality of life through active participation (Totsika *et al.*, 2008). Staff team roles must be clearly identified as being enablers. Too much emphasis on being seen as someone who must do things for people risks the likelihood that people are not given opportunities to use skills and to build upon them to become more independent, thus making it more likely that those skills will be lost. If we always 'do things for people' they may lose the motivation and confidence to do things for themselves even though they may have the potential to continue to do them and to build on these skills to do more for themselves.

Meaningful engagement

Engagement is about an individual being supported to participate in a way that works best for them. It focuses on staff doing things with people, providing whatever support is necessary to ensure the experience of being involved and engaged is successful. This can lead to further opportunities to develop skills, expand choice and control, and increase interactions with others. Engagement needs to be meaningful to the person to have any value. Doing nothing, waiting for others, tasks being done for you, or engaging in behaviours that challenge is unlikely to be meaningful for the person (Beadle-Brown *et al.*, 2017).

 Enabling Capable Environments © Pavilion Publishing and Media Ltd and its licensors 2024.

Engagement can take many different forms. It can be doing something useful and constructive with materials, such as painting, building, cooking and baking. It can be interacting with those around us, like going for a coffee with a friend, attending a concert, or as simple as engaging in a conversation. It can also be taking part in group or community activities such as being a member of a local sports club, going shopping, to the cinema, or being part of a local social group.

Thinking space

Before we examine Person-Centred Active Support further, take some time to think about what good day-to-day support involves. Think about the last activity you supported someone with. What was it? How long did it last?

Now think about your role within that activity. In what ways were you able to promote the following:

- Engagement (How involved was the person? Were they doing or watching?)
- Independence (Was the person able or willing to do things for or by themselves?)
- Choice (Did the person choose what to do? How did they indicate they wanted to finish? Was this respected?)
- Interactions (Was it enjoyable? Were the interactions warm and positive?)

Figure 7.2: Person-Centred Active Support and enhancing quality of life as outlined by Beadle-Brown *et al* (2017).

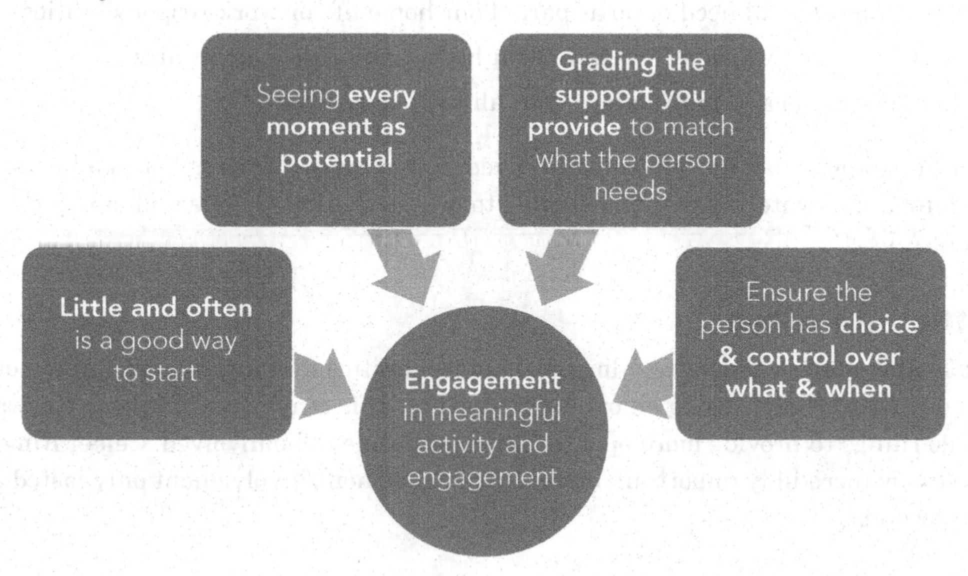

Figure 7.2 shows the four key principles of PCAS and its focus on engagement.

Bigby & Beadle-Brown (2016) have shown evidence of improved quality of life due to staff using PCAS. PCAS is important, at its foundation is the need to promote independence and increase quality of life. This means that in every task and action completed within a supported individual's life, there should be a focus on increasing engagement and participation. This can be achieved by using the four principles of Person-Centred Active Support above.

The four principles of Person-Centred Active Support

There are four core principles of PCAS. These principles help staff teams and those supporting individuals to increase engagement and participation. In this section, we will define each principle before providing an example of how these principles can be applied in practice.

Every moment has potential

The idea that every moment has potential is based on the principle of identifying real and naturally occurring opportunities for engagement, reducing the need to create artificial, tokenistic and limiting activities.

The people we support are surrounded by opportunities for meaningful engagement:

- The things we all need to do as part of our home life or work responsibilities.
- Activities that we enjoy or aspire to at home and in the community.
- Conversations and interactions with all the people around us.

Some examples may include being involved in making a shopping list, reading a book together, watering plants, listening to music, visiting friends and family or exercising.

Little and often

Little and often is about providing many opportunities for engagement throughout the day instead of focusing on one lengthy event. This may mean adapting the way we do things to provide more opportunities for people to be involved. Celebrating success is incredibly important, even if the engagement/involvement only lasted a few seconds.

 Enabling Capable Environments © Pavilion Publishing and Media Ltd and its licensors 2024.

Creating a culture where people can dip in and out of all activities enables engagement at a pace and level that works for the individual. Everything that happens throughout the day is made up of smaller parts or steps. Seeing things this way enables us to identify how people can get involved in the activities and relationships around them.

Thinking about activities and relationships as a series of steps means that we can identify:

- Parts the person can do for themselves.
- Parts we can help them with
- Parts we may need to do for them.

Providing all three parts ensures the person is successful and involved in all aspects of their life.

An example of this principle could be taking time to pinpoint the steps involved in making a cup of tea to identify which parts the person can do themselves, which they need help with, and which parts will need to be done for them. Breaking the entire task into more manageable chunks will allow the person to achieve success and build a skill in a way and at a pace that is right for them. The same principle could also be applied to supporting someone to meet a friend in town, for example.

Graded assistance

People need the right level and type of support at the right time; too much will be over-supported (for example doing things for the person; too little and they may be unsuccessful.

We need to recognise the different types of support each person needs, for example:

- Environmental support – these are things that happen around the activity that help the person understand what to do now or next. The microwave beeps when it finishes, the toast pops when it is done, the light turns green to indicate walking across the road is safe, etc.
- Verbal support – this type of support is spoken information or instructions. This could be someone telling the person the full instructions for a task and letting them do this, it could be providing one step at a time after each previous step is completed, etc. These instructions can be face-to-face, a video recording, etc.

- Visual support – these are gestures, objects, pictures, facial expressions etc. It could be a visual strip with pictures of each step in a full process, or a picture provided as each step is required, it could be another person placing the item required for the next step in front of the person when it is time for that step, or all items being placed in front of the person for the whole task, etc.
- Physical support – this can be direct or indirect physical contact. This may be someone using light physical contact to indicate where to go, indicate where to place something, or more intensive contact to help the person stir a pot, push a button, etc. It is important to remember that touching someone if they do not like this or when they don't expect it is not recommended. Ensure you know the person's preferences and check this regularly.

It is important to note that within each of these types of support, there is a range of levels of support.

We are often too focused on verbal communication and don't appreciate the wealth of non-verbal information people are responding to. In practice, different types and levels of assistance can be used together and staff should switch back and forth between them depending on the person's needs and preferences. If one level of assistance is not working, then staff need to shift to the next level or add a different type so that the person is successful.

Types of assistance

Five types of assistance can support engagement. These are also arranged in a hierarchical structure so less/more support can be provided as required by the person and a drive towards independence can be provided when/if the person is ready for this. Below are the five types structured from the lowest level of support to the highest level of support:

Ask/invite A verbal prompt that suggests to the person that it's time to do something or that something needs to be done.

An example of this might be asking if someone would like to go for a walk. Using this type of assistance would be the right level of support for the person to then, for example, get their jacket, put their shoes on and get their wallet and keys before heading out.

Enabling Capable Environments © Pavilion Publishing and Media Ltd and its licensors 2024.

Instruct A series of verbal prompts that tells the person what to do one step at a time. The person may need help and guidance throughout the activity to achieve this.

An example of this would be 'put the tea bag in the cup'. After this instruction is completed, another instruction would be given, 'pour the water from the kettle into the cup', etc. until the full task is completed.

Prompt A clear gesture or sign to tell the person what to do next. It is like an instruction but works better when the person does not easily understand words.

An example of this would be pointing to the fridge when it is time for the milk to be put away after making tea.

Show This involves demonstrating what needs to be done to another person. You give a demonstration and then the person does the same thing immediately afterwards.

An example of this would be planting a seed in soil and then the other person copying what you have done.

Guide This is providing the person with direct physical assistance to do something. The type of physical support and how long you do it can vary according to the person's needs.

An example of this would be using hand-over-hand support to allow someone to chop vegetables to make dinner.

Maximising choice and control

Choice is an important part of people's lives. Choice should always be encouraged, and the person being supported should be making as many decisions as they feel comfortable making about what they do and when. There are times when we have responsibilities that need to be met such as paying bills, going to work, and putting the bins out for collection, but there are choices within these responsibilities. Most of the time we do get to choose *when*, *where* and *how* we do those tasks. Some examples might be choosing to pay a bill by direct debit so you don't need to go to the bank, for some of us we can work flexibly not 9-5 or it can be more nuanced, to have a bath rather than a shower or completing personal care later in the day

Enabling Capable Environments © Pavilion Publishing and Media Ltd and its licensors 2024.

rather than earlier. Encouraging the person to make choices about what, when, where and how to complete tasks is a core component of PCAS.

If staff frequently respond to preferences expressed by the person they are supporting, the person will learn that there is a point to making choices and will make more of them. By increasing someone's choice you are increasing their control. Look for opportunities to let individuals choose and respect their choices.

Some examples may include when to go shopping, how to contact friends and family (by phone, in person, video call), what to cook for dinner and when to do housework.

Thinking space

Now that we have defined the four principles of PCAS, take some time to think about someone you support. In what ways can you incorporate each principle into the everyday support that you provide?

Use the table below (7.1) and think of some everyday experiences you already do or could introduce to someone you know or support.

Table 7.1: Identifying opportunities for active support

	Principle	Opportunities to develop (In the spaces below identify what the opportunites are and how you will develop these
1	Every moment has potential	
2	Little and often	
3	Graded assistance	
4	Maximising choice and control	

 Enabling Capable Environments © Pavilion Publishing and Media Ltd and its licensors 2024.

When do we need PCAS?

Case study

Consider this example:

You enter the kitchen to see a staff member making the person supported a cup of tea. They do not ask what she wants to drink but, when asked about this, they say they have supported the person for 20 years and they know she always chooses tea and always likes to have it with milk and two sugars. They make it for her at 11 am every time they are on shift because they really care.

Taking what you have learnt so far about PCAS, what are your thoughts on this support?

Think about:

- How involved the person is in the process?
- What choices are available to the person?
- How much assistance is provided?
- How much opportunity is available to the person to become involved?

Consider this next example:

Stephen is a man with a severe intellectual disability. He doesn't use verbal speech often. The other people he lives with leave him alone as he seems not to like noise and fuss. He spends most of his day sitting by the window. When you raise the possibility of Person-Centred Active Support, staff say that they do offer Stephen the chance to do things, but he doesn't want to, and you should respect his choice to sit on his own doing nothing.

Some points to think about:

- What is happening to understand why Stephen does not like noise and what adjustments are in place to address this?
- How are activities presented to Stephen? Does the presentation consider his communication needs?
- What is it about the support that is offered means Stephen appears to not want to be involved?

Consider each of the four principles of active support in your thinking/discussion about why there are barriers to people implementing PCAS in their support of people.

Enabling Capable Environments © Pavilion Publishing and Media Ltd and its licensors 2024.

Barriers to PCAS

Look at the phrases below and think about times when you may have used them or been in a situation when others around you have. Keep these phrases in your mind when you consider the challenging misconceptions section of this chapter.

- 'She's always had it this way for as long as I can remember so she must like it.'
- 'It's easier if I make it as I don't want to upset him.'
- 'It's his choice if he doesn't want to do anything.'
- 'She can't do that so it's better for us both if I do it instead.'

Challenging misconceptions

One of the main barriers for people with intellectual disabilities to be actively involved in activities and experience new opportunities is assumptions made about them by those who support them. Very often people with an intellectual disability are not included and people who support them "do things for the person" rather than support or facilitate their inclusion. Some of these misconceptions include:

- **There is a belief that the more disabled a person is, the less they can do.**

  You can support a better understanding by explaining that individuals may require support to complete certain tasks and activities. Sometimes people need more support, sometimes less. It also depends on what they are doing. You might need to break down activities into smaller pieces and adapt equipment to better meet that person's needs. The key point is that everyone can do some elements, so focus on trying things out and including people.

- **Others may feel they don't want to engage people with complex needs in difficult or long activities in case this causes distress and leads to behaviours that challenge.**

  You can support a better understanding by explaining that we know that behaviours that challenge can be due to boredom and inactivity, therefore support to encourage engagement is essential. You may also explain that we sometimes feel that we cannot support people in some activities or relationships because they are too risky, but our responsibility in these situations is to assess the risk and then manage it appropriately, not eliminate it entirely.

 Enabling Capable Environments © Pavilion Publishing and Media Ltd and its licensors 2024.

- **Support has always happened this way, so it is perceived as working.**

  You can support a better understanding by explaining that just because something has been done one way for a long time, doesn't mean this should continue. People grow and change, and so do preferences and needs. In addition, we know more about how to gain opinions and preferences from those who do not use verbal language. We should ensure their views are being sought as part of the support they receive. The primary outcome of PCAS is engagement in meaningful activities and relationships. It prioritises people doing things for themselves as much as they can over having things done for them. It may have been that, in the past, the way the person was supported to engage in activities was overwhelming or didn't consider their needs and wishes, making the experience aversive and leading to failure. We can change this by utilising the four principles of PCAS and taking these experiences at a pace that is right for the person.

- **If people choose not to engage and participate in activities, this should be respected.**

  You can support a better understanding by explaining that it can be difficult to support people to make informed choices. For people to make choices, they may need support but of more importance, they need the opportunity to make choices and when they do these need to be respected. This support must include information about the different choices available, provided in a format that the person understands. They must also be provided information on what each choice entails as well as the impact of each choice, both positive and negative. For many people, making choices when they have no experience of what is being offered can be daunting. The more we support people to make informed choices the more likely it is they will be confident doing so and supporting teams to understand the ways to promote choice will enhance their confidence in doing this.

- **At times, the person is already busy, or they are too busy to provide this level of support.**

  Studies have found that people with severe intellectual disability typically require support to be involved in meaningful activities (Beadle-Brown *et al.*, 2017: Bigby *et al.*, 2009: Bigby & Beadle-Brown, 2018). If the right support is not provided, they may be left disengaged for the majority of the day which we know results in increased levels of withdrawal, boredom, isolation and behaviours that challenge.

Enabling Capable Environments © Pavilion Publishing and Media Ltd and its licensors 2024.

It is easy to think that people are busy and engaged but the above research has shown that individuals with an intellectual disability particularly those who live in group homes do not receive enough engagement and participation. This research showed that those living in group homes receive only six minutes per hour of assistance from staff to engage in meaningful activities and relationships. Those with the most severe intellectual disability received only one minute per hour. The study found extensive inactivity and isolation among people with severe intellectual disability, even in environments with high staff levels.

Another factor to consider is that those supporting the person are *busy* completing household tasks or organisational-driven tasks such as filling in paperwork for audits, etc. As we discuss in chapter five organisational-driven tasks can be more focused on compliance to meet regulatory body standards, which are critical in-service standards but should not be to the detriment of meeting the needs of the person they are supporting. Staff teams may feel organisational tasks need to be prioritised but it is important to consider whether some of these tasks could be done at different times that do not interfere with support. For those tasks that are a priority, using the four principles of PCAS means the person can be involved in all the tasks.

Inclusion, independence and choice

People with an intellectual disability are entitled to lives which are as full as anyone else's. Although every one of us is different, there are some things we all have in common. In most cases it is important for people to:

- Have relationships that last.
- Have choice and control in their lives.
- Be part of a community.
- Be valued and respected as citizens and treated as an individual.
- Have opportunities to develop experiences and learn new skills.

This is where a PCAS approach is needed. As discussed, PCAS has been found to increase inclusion, independence and choice. Below are some examples of why this is important.

 Enabling Capable Environments © Pavilion Publishing and Media Ltd and its licensors 2024.

- **Inclusion**: Activities and tasks naturally occur throughout the day. PCAS helps to identify and support people to take part in ordinary activities where they have the opportunity to interact with other people.
- **Independence**: PCAS allows people to broaden their experiences by giving just enough help and support for them to experience success. This is hugely important in building, skills, self-worth and self-esteem.
- **Choice**: Ensuring people make choices about their lives and then respecting their decisions will help in broadening their experiences.

Thinking space

Now that we have discussed why PCAS is needed, think about how we plan for this support to happen.

Consider the following:

- Who is responsible for planning the support?
- How is the support organised and allocated?
- Where does planning and allocating of support rank among other service priorities?

Finally, think about someone you currently support. Think about their current levels of engagement and answer the following questions:

- How much time is the person engaged in meaningful activity? What are the high and low spots?
- What is the balance of activities? New/old, exciting/everyday? Different areas of life?
- How many people is the person meeting? How positive are these interactions?

Developing plans and implementing PCAS

Within their training programme, Hume *et al.* (2021) had a particular focus on engagement and participation. The attention was on upskilling frontline managers (trainee practice leaders, see Chapter 6) in their knowledge and understanding of the key elements of PCAS. It is important to note that this process was not simply about training, there was also a real focus on enhancing their skills in applying what had been learnt with their staff teams. The aim of this was to increase the engagement levels of individuals who were being supported within the service and to improve the support offered to staff responsible for implementing the plans.

To support the trainee practice leaders in the implementation of PCAS, the scaffolding approach was used alongside the development and implementation of a Periodic Service Review (see Chapter 5).

Figure 7.3: The Scaffolding Approach: from knowing to doing

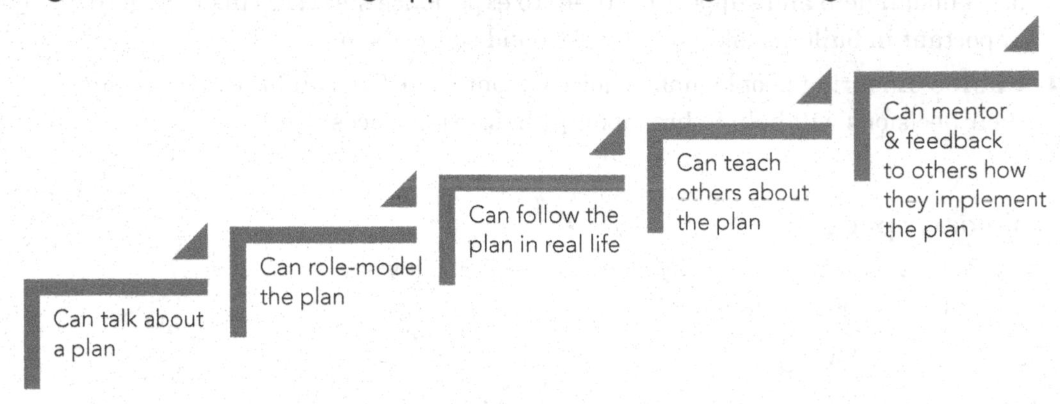

Figure 7.3 shows the scaffolding approach that was used in the Hume *et al*. (2021) programme. This form of scaffolding helps transfer knowledge into practice (i.e. from knowing to doing) and fits with many of the components of practice leadership. It is a systematic process designed to help people transition from being able to say what needs to be done (verbal competence), to being able to describe what they should do and why, to being able to perform those skills in practice where they are needed (practice competence) (LaVigna, 1994).

The initial focus of the programme was on ensuring the trainee practice leaders had a clear and in-depth understanding of the theory underpinning PCAS. This better equipped the trainees to identify opportunities where PCAS could be utilised and provided them with the knowledge to answer questions others had about PCAS (i.e. being able to explain why and how PCAS is effective). As described above, it also provided them with the skills to challenge misconceptions and encourage the staff team to apply the new model of support being implemented. This also allowed the trainees to more effectively role model support and mentor staff in practice.

After gaining this initial knowledge and understanding of PCAS, trainees were asked to identify a focus person and staff team in the service that they would support using PCAS and the scaffolding approach. During the sessions, trainees were supported by the trainers to identify an opportunity for PCAS for their focus person and develop a PCAS plan that could be implemented with them and their

 Enabling Capable Environments © Pavilion Publishing and Media Ltd and its licensors 2024.

team. The plan was based on the four principles of active support and was designed to not only allow the managers to identify areas of focus for each principle but also to identify how and when this plan would be implemented. Below is an example of areas identified by one of the trainees for their focus individual and team.

Person-Centred Active Support planner			
Every moment has potential	**What?**	**How?**	**When?**
Identifying real and naturally occurring opportunities for engagement (reduces the need to create artificial, tokenistic and limiting activities).	With support from his team, Krishnan takes the bus multiple times a week to go shopping, see his family, attend events, etc. (Previously, staff have paid the bus driver for a ticket). Krishnan is now learning how to pay for his own bus ticket.	Prior to leaving the house, Krishnan and his team check he has the correct money to pay for his ticket. When the bus is approaching his support worker reminds him to get his wallet out of his pocket. Krishnan gets on the bus first. Staff should stand near but allow Krishnan to lead the conversation with the driver and to pay.	Every time Krishnan takes the bus.
		If Krishnan says no, staff should reassure him this is okay and then should lead the interaction and get the bus ticket.	

Little and often	What?	How?	When?
Everything that happens throughout the day is made up of smaller parts or steps. Seeing things this way enables us to identify how people can get involved in the activities and relationships available.	Krishnan attends a local badminton group. At the end of the badminton session, everyone goes to the juice bar for a chat. Previously, Krishnan's staff would support him to leave at this point to get the bus as they thought he would find it hard to interact with the group.	At the end of the session, Krishnan's staff will remind him that the juice and chat session is going to take place. They will remind him he can choose if he wants to stay for this. His staff will also remind Krishnan that he can go outside and take a break and come back in if he would like. Staff will show Krishnan where he can go for a break.	Every Thursday after the badminton session
		They should also remind Krishnan that if he wants to leave completely, this is okay and they can go. Krishnan's staff should praise him for any time he stays at the juice and chat session.	

Enabling Capable Environments © Pavilion Publishing and Media Ltd and its licensors 2024.

Graded assistance	What?	How?	When?
People need the right level & type of support at the right time: too much and they will be over-supported, too little and they will be unsuccessful.	Every week Krishnan's friend comes around for pizza night. Previously, Krishnan's staff have made the pizzas and Krishnan has set the table. Using a recipe guide made of pictures Krishnan can now follow the recipe to prepare and cook the pizzas.	Krishnan's picture recipe breaks down the whole task into smaller chunks. For each 'chunk', staff to offer the level of support that Krishnan needs to achieve the task without taking over. (See graded assistance.)	Every pizza night.

Enabling Capable Environments © Pavilion Publishing and Media Ltd and its licensors 2024.

Maximising choice and control	What?	How?	When?
Choice is an important part of people's lives, but for people with an intellectual disability the choice about what they want to do and when or with whom can often be overlooked.	Previously, Krishnan's staff would decide what tasks would be done on what days of the week. This would be completed every Sunday and then shared with Krishnan. Krishnan is now supported to design the next week's planner every Sunday.	A blank visual planner is to be created and shared with Krishnan. All the tasks and activities that need to be completed at set times are to be discussed with Krishnan and added to the board. For all other activities and tasks, Krishnan is to be supported to choose when he would like to do these (i.e. going to the bank, meeting friends, going shopping, going to the cinema, etc.)	The board will be developed every Sunday with Krishnan. It is also reviewed daily based on Krishnan's plans that day.

The inclusion of the columns for 'how' and 'when' encouraged the course participants to think in real terms about what type of support would be required and when this should happen. This was important as it made course participants think about realistic and achievable areas for Person-Centred Active Support for an individual in their service. Once areas were identified using the above template, individual plans were developed for the activities or tasks identified. Not all PCAS opportunities require a plan to be written but there may be some opportunities that you want to encourage and monitor and creating plans alongside a PSR (see Chapter 5) will help to do this. Creating these types of plans helps staff in understanding what they should do in a specific situation.

 Enabling Capable Environments © Pavilion Publishing and Media Ltd and its licensors 2024.

Below is an example of a plan based on an activity that was identified for Krishnan using the planning tool.

PCAS plan for buying my bus ticket

- Before the bus arrives, you should ask Krishnan if he would like to pay for his ticket himself today.
- Remind Krishnan what this entails (for example, having money to pay for the ticket).
- Say 'You will say hello and one return please'. Wait for Krishnan to nod yes to this.
- Then say, 'You will then give your change to the driver'. Again, wait for Krishnan to nod to this.
- Then say, 'You need to take your ticket'. Wait for Krishnan to nod again.
- Ask Krishnan again if he would like to pay for his ticket today.

If he says yes to paying:

- You should help him to get his change ready.
- When the bus arrives, you should allow Krishnan to get on the bus first. You should stand near but allow Krishnan to lead the conversation with the driver and to pay.
- After Krishnan pays and gets his ticket, you should praise him.

If Krishnan struggles and looks to you for support:

- You should step closer and offer reassurance. This may be enough for Krishnan to continue.
- If he is becoming distressed, ask if he would like you to help and do so if he says yes.

If Krishnan says no to wanting to pay for his ticket:

- You should reassure him this is okay and then should lead the interaction and get the bus ticket.
- You can remind Krishnan he can try again another time.

Outcomes of the Hume *et al.* (2021) training initiative

PCAS was a key component of the work undertaken by Hume *et al.* (2021). We know engagement and participation levels are usually low when supporting people with higher support needs (Bigby *et al.*, 2009, Bigby & Beadle-Brown., 2018), the trainers of this programme collected data using the active support measure (ASM) to ascertain levels of current support and engagement.

The ASM (Mansell *et al.*, 2005) is a 15-question assessment tool that measures the engagement and participation of individuals and the skill with which staff provide and support these opportunities. Each question is scored from 0 to 3, with 0 being poor support to 3 being good, skilled support. The maximum score using this measure is 45. Some examples of questions asked are about the choice of activities, staff working as a team and interpersonal warmth.

The reason for using the ASM within the pilot programme is that it not only looks at whether support is being provided but more importantly the quality of that support. Within their pilot programme, Hume *et al.* (2021) completed six observations using the ASM. An average score was taken before the implementation of PCAS plans. Follow-up observations involved a further ASM per person throughout the training programme and again after the completion of the training programme.

Figure 7.4: Active Support Measure Score

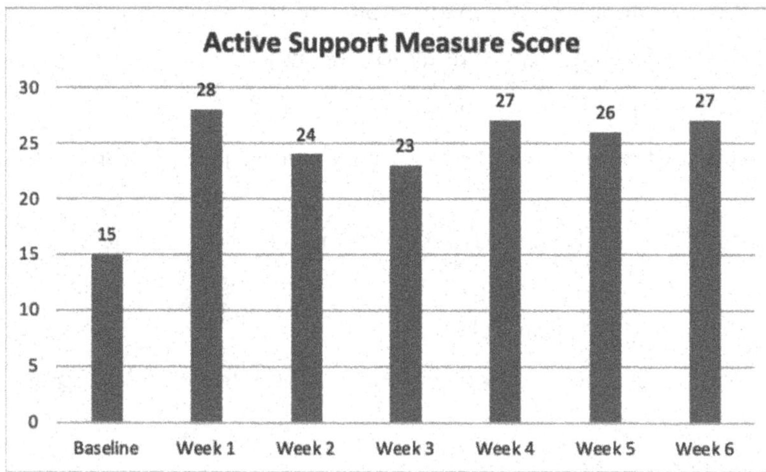

Figure 7.4 shows the ASM scores for one of the focus individuals throughout the training. The graph shows the increase in ASM scores throughout the training programme's implementation, including the implementation of the ten-a-day observations (discussed in more detail in Chapter 2 and Chapter 5). The graph shows increased ASM scores throughout the training programme when compared to scores before the training programme's implementation. The graph also shows

Enabling Capable Environments © Pavilion Publishing and Media Ltd and its licensors 2024.

that scores do not lower to the level achieved during baseline data capture. The data shows that while the ten-a-day was being implemented, scores for the ASM increased and stayed above the baseline scores (before implementation).

Factors that support PCAS

Several factors are crucial to the implementation of PCAS. These include:

- The provision of **coaching and mentoring**. As stated previously, practice leadership (see Chapter 6) was provided initially by the trainers to develop the practice leadership skills of the trainees. This was essential as organisational focus tends to be on administrative duties which leads to managers being less visible and not having time to focus on the quality of the support being provided. Trainees were supported in their daily practice by the trainers to be present and directly observe support practices, both focusing on PCAS plans but also general PCAS elements in practice. They were also supported by trainers to provide direct in-person support and guidance to staff, skilling these frontline managers to take this forward within their services.
- Creating a **shared vision**. This was a key focus in ensuring that the trainees understood and were able to carry out the plan. The role of practice leaders must function to communicate a shared vision about what they want to create within a service. Shifting the culture from a focus on reducing challenging behaviour to a focus on quality of life needs strong leadership and teamwork. This is a hugely important step in implementing a collaborative process between managers and staff.
- **Appraising and evaluating** support practices. The continued focus on PCAS was supported through the PSR. In their work, Hume *et al.* (2021) developed a specific PSR standard that focused on PCAS and its implementation. Once managers had identified PCAS opportunities and developed individual plans, a PSR standard was developed to support implementation and evaluate how well the plans were being implemented. This allowed trainees to include PCAS in their observations when carrying out their role as practice leaders. It also ensured that PCAS was integrated into daily support in a meaningful way and that staff and frontline managers were able to visually evaluate progress over time. An example of the PSR standard and template for Krishnan developing his weekly planner is shown below. For full details on how to identify and complete a PSR, see Chapter 5.

Table 7.2: Example of a PSR standard	
What (needs to happen)	Supporting Krishnan to develop his weekly planner.
When (does it happen)	Every Sunday evening.
Who (needs to be involved)	The person supporting Krishnan on Sunday evening. They should complete the corresponding recording tool.
How (Would you know it has happened)	Either: The practice leader observes the planner being developed with Krishnan on Sunday. Or The Practice Leader reviews the recording form that details how well the plan was implemented.

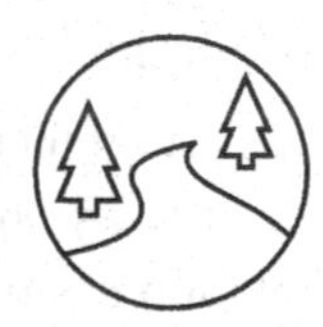

Paving the way to success

Below are some possible questions you are likely to be asked or you will ask during the process of implementing Person-Centred Active Support:

1. **Can PCAS be used with people who have severe intellectual disabilities?**

   Absolutely. You might need to break down activities into smaller pieces and adapt equipment, but PCAS is for everyone, it is a person-centred approach to providing support in a way that the person needs.

2. **It is hard to think of new things to do with the person. Any suggestions?**

   If the individual uses verbal language or has a communication system in place you can ask them for ideas. Additionally, speak to your team, the person's family members and friends to discover what they like to do. Think about the everyday tasks you do at home that they can be involved in. Understand the importance of finding out about the person's history,

 Enabling Capable Environments © Pavilion Publishing and Media Ltd and its licensors 2024.

preferences, wishes and needs, and recognise that everything you do is based on them. People can have great plans but rubbish lives! Person-Centred Active Support works well with other person-centred approaches such as Person-Centred plans, PCAS can help turn Person-Centred Plans into Person-Centred actions by ensuring support is focused on what the person wants and needs.

3. **What if the person says no?**

   It is OK for people to say no but if this happens all the time then you might need to think about how activities and new ideas are presented to the person. Are they presented in a way the person understands, are they activities the person wants to do, are they offered at a time the person would want to do them, etc?

Conclusion

- Person-Centred Active Support is a model of how staff should interact and support people with an intellectual disability and is particularly important for people with high support needs.
- Person-Centred Active Support aims to enhance the quality of life of individuals by providing more opportunities to be fully involved and in control of all aspects of their lives. A key philosophy of PCAS is the shift from a focus on reducing behaviours that challenge to a focus on improving quality of life.
- It concentrates on promoting engagement and participation. We know, people with high support needs spend the majority of their time disengaged or as passive observers. We also know that this can lead to higher levels of withdrawal and isolation, and more frequent engagement in behaviours that challenge.
- Practice leadership is an important part of implementing Person-Centred Active Support in a service setting. Support staff must see their role as enablers rather than carers. Practice leadership is important in ensuring that services are focused on people rather than tasks. It also leads to a collaborative process between managers and staff teams.
- Good support doesn't just happen, it must be planned for (Mansell, 2007), and the staff responsible for implementing this need training and leadership support to do this. Adopting a PCAS framework ensures that supported individuals are the focus of all tasks/activities that have an impact on their lives.

Chapter 8: Enabling Opportunities and Developing New Skills

'Associate yourself repeatedly with a wide variety of activities, people and things the person values, then eventually your presence will become a signal that many rewarding events and activities are available with you.'
Carr *et al*. (1994, p112)

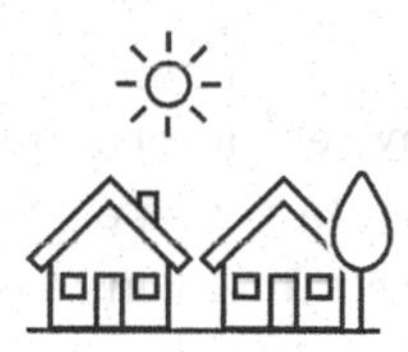

Chapter contents:

- Developing and enabling opportunities for learning new skills for people with an intellectual disability.
- Principles which support teaching and learning.
- The different methods of teaching and the learning styles of people who are acquiring new skills.
- The role of good support planning in the context of learning and teaching.

Learning outcomes

After reading this chapter and completing the suggested activities and reflections, the reader should be able to:

- Understand what is meant by developing skills and opportunities and how this links to quality of life.
- Recognise different teaching approaches and principles and how they are used to support learning and development.

- Identify steps to understanding how to present opportunities to teach and develop new skills.
- Identify the steps to ensure opportunities to learn and use these skills in practice.
- Appreciate how skill development leads to autonomy and independence.

Introduction

Many of us value the opportunity to try new experiences. Some of these opportunities are taken in pursuit of what we would commonly refer to as hobbies. We also pursue new opportunities, not simply to engage in the activity, but also to share interests with people or to meet new people. Other reasons are to become better at something, perhaps for our work, family, or just because it makes us feel good.

From a young age, we are driven by self-determination, and we strive to learn how to do things and to be independent. Have you ever tried to put a two-year-old into a car seat? Up to a certain day, it's all fine; you place them in and fasten the straps. Then, one day, as you try to put them into the seat, they straighten up so you cannot place them in the seat, and they shout, 'Do it myself'. This is wonderful – a child being self-determined – but today you are running late for school and the last thing you need is a self-determined child who doesn't really know how to fasten the straps on the car seat!

So, what do we do? Well, we create learning opportunities, and we promote teaching to empower this self-determination and enhance the person's skills in the context of their quality of life. We also do this naturally, consistently thinking about what skills and opportunities would help the person have a better life. We take the time to teach in a way and at a pace that works for the person (not at a time when you are late for the school run). This is particularly important for people with an intellectual disability as, historically, the concept of providing opportunities for teaching and learning was often not even considered. Regrettably, it was often believed that people with an intellectual disability could not or would not want to learn. We must flip this narrative to examine whether we need to change how we teach.

 Enabling Capable Environments © Pavilion Publishing and Media Ltd and its licensors 2024.

Maximising opportunities

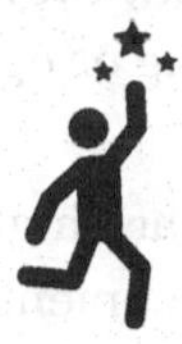

In Chapter 7, we discuss how to maximise opportunities for people with an intellectual disability to be involved in all the daily aspects of their lives, promoting choice and control and doing this in a way that enhances their quality of life. Many of these concepts are also embedded in several person-centred approaches such as person-centred planning, Intensive Interaction, education, health, and care plans, and SEN or EHCP support plans. The tools/plans are specifically designed to find out what is important to a person and the support they need.

There is an abundance of research showing that people with an intellectual disability (more so for adults with an intellectual disability than children) spend a significant amount of time not engaging in activities, not doing things that are meaningful to them or not having the opportunity to pursue friendships and relationships with people they choose (Bigby *et al*., 2009; Bigby & Beadle-Brown, 2018).

There can be several reasons for this:

- People with an intellectual disability tend to be more isolated, so they may not have the social connections to establish relationships. They may live far away from their family and friends and experience restricted travel options. They may live and socialise only with others receiving support or with whom they have little in common.
- People with an intellectual disability may not have access to resources or funds to pursue new interests or hobbies.
- Services restrict people's access to items or locations. For example, environments do not have items the person can use, items may be locked away due to a perceived risk, or the person is not supported to access community-based activities or venues.
- Teams do not know how to engage with the people they are supporting or do not see the value of self-determination.

- There is a lack of aspiration by others to want to support the person with an intellectual disability to achieve what they want to achieve and do what they wish to do, for example skill teaching or opportunities are limited to household tasks.
- Teams may believe it is unfair to place high expectations on the person or that it is too difficult to support skill development.
- The role of support workers and other supporting roles are not given the professional recognition they should have, for example job adverts that state 'all you need are good values' and which fail to recognise that support roles are highly skilled roles. This lack of professional recognition can lead to inadequate training and support being given to staff.

In Chapter 7, we explored that good lives do not just happen; they must be planned. The same concept also applies to creating opportunities for learning and developing – it doesn't just happen; preparation and planning are required. People do not always learn new skills through traditional and outdated teaching methods such as repetition or being told what to do or not to do. Teaching new skills is not a one-size-fits-all approach. It needs to tap into what the person wants to learn and their learning style, so we must consider our teaching style. People are more likely to learn when they are interested in the activity or task, when it serves a purpose for them, the learning process is fun and exciting, and they are being taught by someone they like or alongside people they like.

Learning new skills

Learning new things is inherent to us. We strive to improve at the things we enjoy, things which will help us in our work, or to get a better job, or that will allow us to spend time doing things with people we like. We also learn new skills in order to be independent and self-determined (see chapters 1, 7 and 10). In our experience, plans for teaching skills to people with an intellectual disability centre around self-care tasks or household tasks. These are fundamental skills to have, but, in many ways, if this is all we are teaching people, it can lead to a very empty and dull existence.

 Enabling Capable Environments © Pavilion Publishing and Media Ltd and its licensors 2024.

So, what do we teach?

An excellent place to start is with skills the person would want to learn or skills that might improve their quality of life. There may be goals or aspirations in the person's plan, for example in:

- Their person-centred plan.
- Their circles of support person-centred planning tool.
- Their relationships circle person-centred planning tool.

You might also identify opportunities for learning and development as part of:

- A capable environments appraisal (Chapter 2).
- The person's IEP (Individual Education Plan).
- Their Multi-Element Behaviour Support Plan (Chapter 10).
- Their sensory profile or health assessment (Chapters 2 and 3).
- An appraisal of the quality-of-life domains (Chapter 1).

Think about what is helpful to or preferred by the person:

- Learning a fun skill.
- Learning a practical skill.
- Learning a communication skill.
- Learning how to make a complaint about their support.
- Learning how to cope in a difficult situation (if that situation cannot be avoided, for example, the bus breaking down).

When teaching new skills or supporting new opportunities:

- Be engaging with the person, use their name and be genuine in your interest in them and the activity.
- Think about the environment, how can it be set up to maximise success? (i.e. having all items at hand, little distractions, spaces to break away from the task for a short while, etc.)
- Be consistent, but also flexible to the person's needs and learning style.
- Use visual prompts.
- Use role modelling.

Enabling Capable Environments © Pavilion Publishing and Media Ltd and its licensors 2024.

- Think about when and where learning a new skill will happen.
- Think about ways to learn a new skill, this can be:
  - one to one
  - as part of play
  - in real life
  - with peers

Principles to support teaching

We will explore several teaching methods later in this chapter, but many share fundamental principles. These principles include:

1. How to understand the task being taught, for example by breaking down the sequence into steps, also known as *task analysis*.
2. Considering how each of the steps may be best taught, for example teaching each step from the beginning of the sequence (*forward chaining*) or teaching from the last step of the sequence (*backward chaining*).
3. Finally, matching your behaviour to the person's learning style. This includes thinking about how you support learning by using *prompts/reinforcement*.

Task Analysis

Task analysis involves breaking down a task into smaller, more manageable steps to support teaching and learning. The principle is to teach each of the steps until the person can complete the entire task. This can look different depending on the activity being taught and the skills and learning needs of the person. An example of a task analysis is provided in Table 8.1 later in this chapter.

It is important when creating a task analysis that all steps within the task are considered. There are different ways to achieve this:

 Enabling Capable Environments © Pavilion Publishing and Media Ltd and its licensors 2024.

1. You could think about a specific task and note down all the steps involved, then work through these one by one to complete the task and identify if any steps are missing.
2. You could watch another person doing the task and note down the steps involved.
3. You could bring a group of people together to consider the steps required.

Thinking space

Think about a task you complete every day. What are the steps involved in achieving it? Using Figure 8.2 as a guide, create a task analysis for this activity.

Now go further and think about someone you support doing this task. What steps would be needed for them to achieve this task as independently as possible?

- Are the steps the same as your own task analysis?
- How many new skills would they need to learn to achieve the task?

After completing a task analysis, you now need to consider the best way to teach this skill. Below are two examples of chaining methods that may support learning.

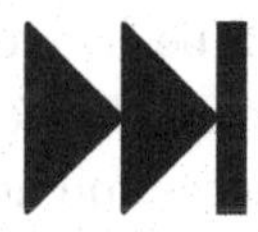

Forward chaining

Forward chaining is a way of teaching the steps of a task analysis in the order in which the task/activity occurs. Only one step is taught at a time, starting with the first step in the task analysis. Once the person can complete the first step of the chain independently, you then work on teaching (and reinforcing) the second step. For example, if you are teaching a person to put on a t-shirt, you may start by just teaching them to put it on their head. The person teaching would then praise the person and remind them how well they have done before completing all the subsequent steps. Once the person can put the t-shirt on their head independently, you may work on teaching them to place the t-shirt on their head and then pull it down to their neck. This continues advancing one step at a time until all task analysis steps are completed independently. This type of teaching is helpful when

Enabling Capable Environments © Pavilion Publishing and Media Ltd and its licensors 2024.

a person may have difficulty learning multiple steps at once, and relatively easy steps are needed at the beginning. The benefit of this approach to chaining is that it minimises frustration for the learner and increases their likelihood of success.

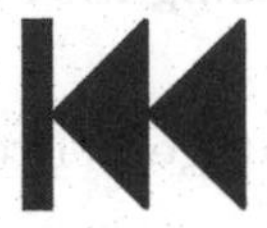

Backward chaining

Backward chaining is a way of teaching the steps of a task one step at a time, but this time starting with the final step. For example, in a backwards chain of ten steps, the person teaching would complete the first nine steps and work on teaching the person to complete the final step independently. Once that step is mastered, the person works on steps nine and ten. For example, when making a cake, the last step may be for the person to put the fruit on the top. Once a person can do this independently, they would be taught the previous step of putting the cream on the sponge and then the fruit on top. This continues, moving backwards one step at a time until all task analysis steps are completed independently. This type of teaching is helpful when learning multiple steps at once, and the end of the chain results in something that the person likes (e.g., eating cake).

After deciding which chaining method best meets the person's needs and preferences, it is important to consider the type of support that will be provided to ensure the person successfully completes the new skill.

Prompting or guiding

Prompts and guides are supportive strategies that those teaching new skills can use to help a person complete a task or steps in a task. Below are some examples of prompts and guides that can be used:

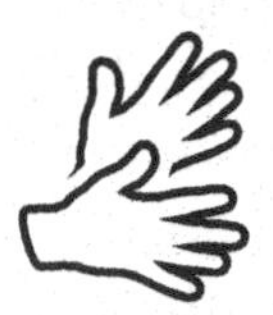

Physical prompts: These involve using physical contact to support a person to complete a task (i.e. placing the person's hand on the knife and gently holding it there while cutting a slice of cake; placing the person's hand over the teacher's hand when stirring a pot; directing the learner to put the key in the door through gentle touch and movement to the person's elbow, etc.).

Enabling Capable Environments © Pavilion Publishing and Media Ltd and its licensors 2024.

Verbal prompt: These are verbal statements or instructions that indicate what the person should do (i.e. press the button, get the spoon, walk to the table, etc.).

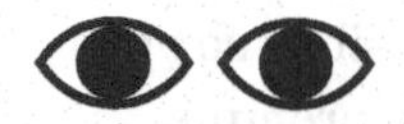

Modelling prompt: These prompts involve doing the task first and then showing the person to do it (i.e. stir the pot and then the person stirs the pot; place your hand in the position of the guitar chord and then the person can copy this; do a few steps in dance routine and the person copies and joins in, etc.)

Positional prompt: These involve placing items closest to the person to indicate they are the next item that will be required.

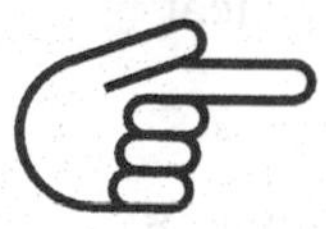

Gestural prompt: These prompts provide physical movements from the teacher that indicate what to do next (i.e. pointing to an item, walking towards an area, nodding towards the next item required, etc.).

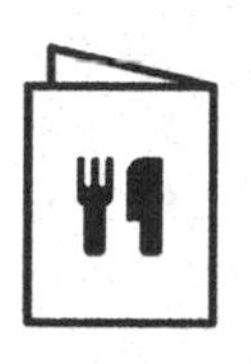

Visual prompt: These are visual prompts in the person's environment to support them to complete a task. They might be a list of instructions in a set order, a recipe, a calendar, etc. These can be in written, visual, or pictorial form that the person follows independently.

Deciding what prompts to use depends on the activity and the person's learning style (Beadle-Brown *et al.*, 2017). The main aim is to support the person to be as independent as possible. Therefore, considering how to fade out (reduce and remove) prompts as the person becomes more independent is important. The prompts above are listed in order of most supportive to most independent. For example, you may begin with a physical and verbal prompt, reduce it to just a physical prompt, and finally be able to have no prompts. If you need to re-introduce prompts if the person is getting stuck, then it is OK to do this. The prompts used will depend on the person and their needs. Some people may need all prompts and combinations of prompts, while others may only need two or three of the techniques.

It is important to note that some prompts may not be right for some individuals. For instance, some people may not like physical contact, so avoiding this prompt would be essential. Other people may not like verbal language, so ensuring another type of prompt would be necessary.

Enabling Capable Environments © Pavilion Publishing and Media Ltd and its licensors 2024.

It is also essential to consider the person's learning style and previous experiences of learning new skills. You may decide to start with the most supportive strategies as the person has experienced previous failures when learning new skills, and therefore you do not want them to experience any lack of success. On the other hand, you may support someone who likes to be as independent as possible, so you start with the most independent prompt and only use more supportive prompts when required to ensure success.

As an example, we will use a scenario in which Jake is learning to download some music from an online music provider. In this example, we start with the least level of prompting as Jake likes to try new things. For Jake, his most independent prompt is a gestural prompt which moves to a more supportive level of prompting (modelling), and then the most supportive prompting Jake requires (a physical prompt).

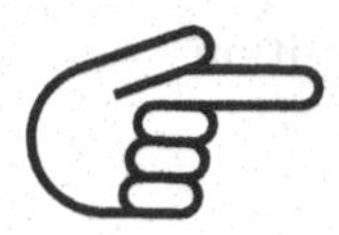

Gestural prompt: You point to the download button on Jakes's device. Perhaps also miming your finger pressing the 'download' button

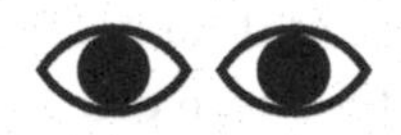

Modelling prompt: you have the same piece of equipment as Jake, so you show him on your device how to press 'download'.

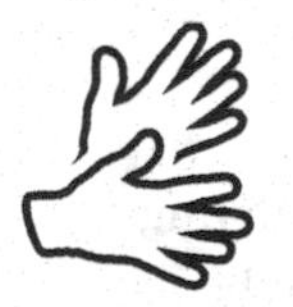

Physical prompt: direct physical hand-over-hand support to complete the action.

As the person is learning each of the steps, prompts should be followed with a clear message that the person is doing well (*reinforcement*). This may be something like a positive comment, such as 'well done', a high five or thumbs up, or it could be that the step of the activity is motivating/reinforcing in itself, for example, the last step of making a cake is to eat it!

Methods or ways of teaching

Now that you are aware of some of the key principles of teaching, we will consider some of specific teaching methods.

So, how do we teach new skills? There are several teaching philosophies and approaches we can use. Here, we will explain some of these approaches, which

 Enabling Capable Environments © Pavilion Publishing and Media Ltd and its licensors 2024.

can be applied in several settings, such as the person's home or in the classroom. We will explore three of these with examples in this chapter.

- Collaborative approach.
- Direct instruction.
- Active learning.

Collaborative approach

A collaborative (or cooperative) learning approach involves people/students working together on activities or learning tasks in a group small enough to ensure that everyone can participate (Laal & Laal, 2012). People/students in the group may work on separate tasks that contribute to a common overall outcome, or they might work together to support one student to complete tasks that benefit the group. It is also an approach that considers the skills a person already has and focusses on expanding them. This is also referred to as **Vygotsky's Scaffolding Approach** (Figure 8.1). It supports a learn-by-doing approach and working with others.

Figure 8.1: Vygotsky's scaffolding approach

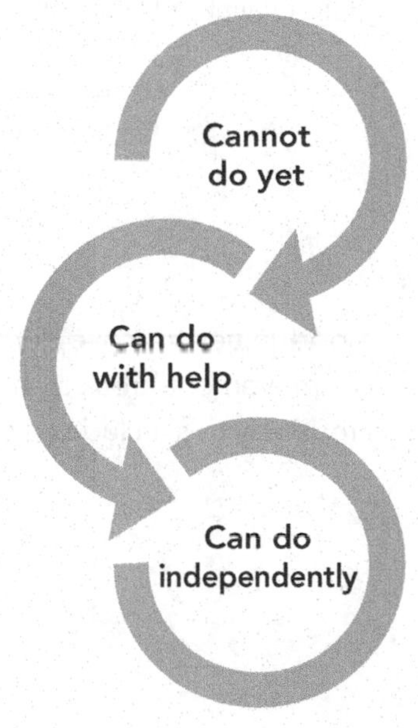

Enabling Capable Environments © Pavilion Publishing and Media Ltd and its licensors 2024.

In this model, a person's level of ability falls into one of three categories:

- The person can do a task themselves: independently without assistance.
- The person can do part of a task: they need support or direction to complete it.
- The person cannot do a task: they have not had the experience to learn this skill.

The principle of this approach is that the 'teacher' scaffolds what is being taught. This is done by identifying what the person can do and what they cannot do. The parts they cannot do are broken down into smaller chunks to teach. In principle, the idea is to move through each of the parts of the scaffold in a way that works for the learner. The advantages to learning and teaching of a scaffolding approach are that it does not assume the person knows nothing; they are not a blank canvas. It acknowledges that most of the time people already have skills that can be applied to at least part of a task, and therefore it builds on these existing skills.

The case study below illustrates how this scaffolding approach enhances collaborative learning.

Case study: Sam

Sam is five years old, and her sensory profile shows that she needs regular movement breaks (proprioceptive feedback). In her classroom setting, these can happen as part of a group activity and with peer learning – for example, at break time, a variety of activities to promote movement are available to all children including games and activities such as:

- Parachute game.
- Skipping.
- Trampoline.
- An activity circuit for teams.

However, Sam may also need opportunities to move during class time, Sam does not always recognise that she needs a movement break so her teachers have thought of ways to have movement breaks routinely this includes a skill that Sam could learn to help with this.

 Enabling Capable Environments © Pavilion Publishing and Media Ltd and its licensors 2024.

Skill: handing out workbooks for her class table (Figure 8.2).

- At the beginning of a session, Sam's teacher asks her to help hand out the books for the other five students at Sam's table.
- Sam's teacher gathers the six books needed and goes to the table of students, if Sam doesn't follow, her teacher can say again 'Can you help me with the books, Sam?'
- Sam's teacher places a book in front of one child and says, 'Book one for Charlie' (Sam loves counting, so this will help engage her with the task).
- The teacher then moves to the next child: 'Book two for Jake', and so on.
- At the last child, Sam's teacher gives Sam the book and points to Karla saying, 'book five for Karla' while handing the book to Sam.
- Sam's teacher thanks her for her help and the students give Sam a round of applause.

As Sam becomes more confident, her teacher will move to asking Sam to hand out the last two books, and then the last three, until Sam can independently hand out all of the books for her table.

In this scenario, Sam is only asked to hand out the last book (the last part of the task). This is an example of *backwards chaining*, discussed earlier. It also gives Sam the opportunity to see what the task is – her teacher has handed out the first four books, so she is *modelling* the task. It builds on a skill Sam is good at and likes (counting), it helps meet her sensory needs in a *functional* way, and the other students can *collaborate* in the activity to ensure success.

Written activity plans are essential to ensure those who are teaching the new skills do so consistently. It also means the learner is able to practice and follow steps in a way that is predictable for them, and that the plan is personalised to their learning style. Having a written plan means it is possible to see how progress is being made, for example the person is learning all of the steps of the skill. It also allows you to identify whether the plan needs to be reviewed, for example if the person is getting stuck at the same stage then this would suggest the plan may need to be broken down into smaller steps.

Figure 8.2: Sample activity plan for Sam using a collaborative learning approach

The activity

Handing out workbooks at beginning of lesson at 11am each day

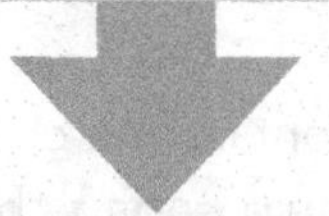

Why this activity

Sam needs activities to encourage her to move from her table several times a day

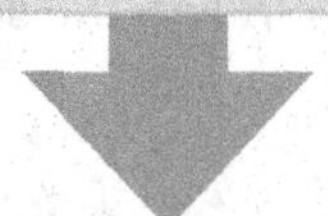

Setting up the activity

1) Get books at correct time 2) Ask Sam to help give out books	1) Teacher does this stage 2) Teacher stands next to the table and verbally asks Sam to hand a book to a student

Parts of activity	Prompts (from students and teacher)	Praise (this is from the students and the teacher)
Handing out book one to Charlie	Students may respond to their name by putting their hand up. The teacher stands next to the table and gives Sam one book at a time saying, 'This book is for *insert name*'. The teacher may prompt by pointing to the student.	Students and teacher may respond with: 'Well done, Sam.' 'Thank you, Sam.' 'Great work Sam.' 'You are doing a fantastic job.'
Handing out book two to Jake		
Handing out book three to Karla		
Handing out book four to Lia		
Handing out book five to Alex		
Giving Sam her book	Verbal prompt to Sam.	

 Enabling Capable Environments © Pavilion Publishing and Media Ltd and its licensors 2024.

Direct instruction

Direct instruction is a more directed teaching method. In this method, we want to teach each specific step of a task in a sequence and reinforce is so that the person can move to completing the task independently.

This means that the person teaching presents the information or decides the steps in a task based on how the task or activity should be done. It is more of an explicit, guided instruction to the person learning the task/activity (Donnellan *et al.*, 1988). An example of this could be teaching someone the steps of an activity using a **task analysis** approach with clear instructions and reinforcement at each stage. An example of this might be learning how to set a table for dinner.

Case study: Felix

Felix has recently moved into a house with two other people. He finds it difficult to wait, and while he does have some support such as a timer and a now and next board, there are times when these supports are not enough. For example, there are some days when everyone has dinner together and take turns cooking.

On these days, just before dinner Felix tries to hurry people to the table and becomes annoyed when they do not. The people who he lives with are also becoming annoyed with Felix as they do not like to be rushed. To fill a gap in his support, Felix's support team think he could learn a new skill (setting the table), which could bridge the gap of time and give him an opportunity to do something independently and not feel he needs to rush his housemates.

Enabling Capable Environments © Pavilion Publishing and Media Ltd and its licensors 2024.

Below is an example of an activity plan that has been created to support Felix in setting the table using direct instruction.

<table>
<tr><th colspan="4">Table 8.1: Sample activity plan using task analysis</th></tr>
<tr><td colspan="4">Teaching skills to set the table</td></tr>
<tr><td colspan="4">Purpose of plan: to learn a new skill – to set the table; to develop an independent skill; to help Felix fill some time before dinner.</td></tr>
<tr><td colspan="4">Setting up the environment:
■ Support worker to place the following on the worktop next to the cooker from left to right and in the following order.
  ■ Five mats.
  ■ Five plates – stacked on top of each other.
  ■ Five knives.
  ■ Five forks.
  ■ Five glasses – stacked on top of each other.
■ This activity will happen at 5.30 on each day everyone is eating together.
■ Individual support is to be provided for this activity.</td></tr>
<tr><td colspan="4">Steps of the activity</td></tr>
<tr><td>Step</td><td>Teaching prompt
(What staff will do)</td><td>Actions
(What Felix will do)</td><td>Reinforcing outcome</td></tr>
<tr><td>1. Bring the placemats</td><td>Point to the mats then Verbal prompt – 'take the mats to the table'.
Gestural prompt towards the table.</td><td>Takes the mats to the table.</td><td rowspan="2">Correct responses
'Thanks, that was good.
'Well done, Felix!'<br>'You're doing great.'</td></tr>
<tr><td>2. Lay the placemats</td><td>Verbal prompt – 'Place a mat here'.
Gestural prompt – point to the area for each mat to be placed.</td><td>Place one mat at each end of the table and one in the middle.</td></tr>
</table>

Enabling Capable Environments © Pavilion Publishing and Media Ltd and its licensors 2024.

3. Bring the knives	Point to the mats then **Verbal prompt** – 'Take the knives to the table' & **Gestural prompt** towards the table.	Takes the knives to the table.	
4. Lay the knives	**Verbal prompt** – 'Place a knife here'. **Gestural prompt** – point to the area for each knife to be placed.	Place a knife to the right side of each mat.	
5. Bring the forks	Point to the forks then **Verbal prompt** – 'Take the forks to the table'. **Gestural prompt** towards the table.	Takes the forks to the table.	**Incorrect responses** Repeat **verbal prompt**. Increase to **gestural prompt** then a physical prompt if needed.
6. Lay the forks	**Verbal prompt** – 'Place a fork here'. **Gestural prompt** – point to the area for each fork to be placed.	Place a fork to the left of each mat.	
7. Bring the glasses	Point to the glasses then **Verbal prompt** – 'Take the glasses to the table'. **Gestural prompt** towards the table.	Takes the glasses (stacked) to the table.	
8. Lay the glasses	**Verbal Prompt** – 'Place a glass here'. **Gestural prompt** – point to the area for each glass to be placed.	Place a glass at the top of each mat.	

Communication style and prompts

- Staff to use a fun and upbeat tone of voice to encourage Felix to participate.
- Staff to go with Felix to the kitchen, still encouraging and being upbeat.
- Staff to stand to the left of Felix, which will ensure you do not get in Felix's way or distract him. It also ensures you are close enough to provide physical prompts when required.
- At the end of the activity, if the table has been set, staff should directly refer to the table and say to Felix, 'Well done, you did that! Let's call the others for dinner'.

Reinforcers – supporting a good outcome

- Felix is more likely to respond if it is clear what is expected of him.
- Felix likes structure and routine. Presenting this activity as described above will keep him focused.
- At the end of the activity, it will be time to call the others and sit for dinner.
- Telling Felix how well he is doing.

Problem solving

Felix may drop an item:

- Staff should pick up the item quickly and place it back in his hand reassuring and encouraging him to keep going, and point to where you want Felix to lay the item.

Felix may refuse to come to the kitchen:

- Ask Felix a second time, following which take one of the items of cutlery to Felix and show him it and state the key phrase: 'Felix, it's time to lay the table'.

Someone may enter the room:

- Keep focused on Felix and the activity. If possible, discreetly ask the other person to wait or leave.

Felix may become focused on one item and get stuck:

- In a clear tone, state, 'Felix, put the (name item) here', and then point to where it needs to go.

Felix may start shouting for you to do it instead:

- In a bright, enthusiastic voice, tell Felix how well he is doing and offer to help so he can move onto the next stage.

Felix may leave the room:

- Wait for him, he sometimes needs a moment or two and usually comes back to an activity after a short break.

Enabling Capable Environments © Pavilion Publishing and Media Ltd and its licensors 2024.

Thinking space

Identify a skill for teaching: what you are teaching and why?

Complete a task analysis – you can find an example in the setting the table plan above.

Decide on the teaching methods you will use and how you will support learning.

Consider how each step will be presented/taught.

Consider what prompts will help and how to fade these out.

Consider the type of feedback (reinforcement) that will help with learning.

Consider what opportunities the person will have to use these new skills.

Active learning

Active learning is a student/learner-centred approach in which the students/learners are more responsible for the direction of learning, and they work collaboratively towards a common goal. It focuses on the students/learners' skills to work out ways to solve problems or achieve tasks, rather than the teacher being seen as the expert who reveals the correct way to do something (Revell & Ayotte, 2020). An example of this is person-centred active support, or practising skills with feedback. Some examples are provided in Chapter 7. Below is an example of teaching Josh to learn how to develop a picture schedule using the principles of active learning.

Learning how to add to a picture schedule using active learning

Why this activity?

- To help Josh to understand what is happening over the specified period of time.
- To help Josh understand what task or activity he is about to do.
- To help Josh anticipate events.
- To help Josh focus on a task or activity.
- To help Josh move from one activity to another.
- To help Josh develop independence.
- To help Josh understand time, routine and expectations.
- To help Josh make choices.

Table 8.2: An example of an activity plan to learn how to make a picture schedule (visual timetable)

Name: Josh

Plan: Picture Schedule

Date: December 2023

Objective: The purpose of the picture schedule is to provide structure to Josh's day. A schedule strip representing three activities or tasks at a time will help Josh predict the next few activities and give his parents a mechanism to encourage his participation.

When to do it: The picture schedule should be completed two or more times daily and the schedule should be followed and referred to throughout the day.

Materials needed:

1. Photos or line drawings of daily activities. It may be helpful to have a typed description of the activity at the bottom of the photo or line drawing. Each picture has Velcro on the back to attach to the schedule strip.
2. A schedule strip that has room for all the photos of all possible activities. Three strips of Velcro will be on the schedule strip.
3. An 'All Done' envelope for pictures representing completed activities/tasks.

Steps:

Step 1. For each activity that might occur during the day, take a photograph/icon representing some portion of that activity (e.g., trampoline, washing dishes, going for a walk, etc.). A master set of all photographs may be stored in a large photo album.

Step 2. At the beginning of each day, look through Josh's photographs with him and take out three pictures representing three tasks/activities which are to be completed next. As much choice as possible should be given to the activity and the order in which they are to be completed. There may be some activities that have set times and/or days but others that can be altered or moved based on preference.

Step 3. The sequence of the three upcoming activities must be reviewed and agreed by Josh. The pictures representing each activity should be selected, and Josh should be included in placing the activity pictures on the schedule strips. It is important that the preferred and less/non-preferred activities be interspersed with each other. Give Josh a high five and tell him he has done well in planning his next activities.

Enabling Capable Environments © Pavilion Publishing and Media Ltd and its licensors 2024.

Step 4. Before starting each activity, Josh should review his schedule. Verbally cue him that it is time to check the schedule, e.g., 'OK, let's go see what we have to do next'. **OR** 'Let's go see what is on your schedule'. He should be encouraged to point to the picture to verbalise the activity and initiate the process.

Step 5. Once the task or activity has been completed, Josh should again be reminded to check his schedule. Josh should remove the picture of the completed task and place it in the 'All Done' envelope.

Step 6. He should then move to the next picture and the process should be repeated. When the three activities on the strip are completed, the next three should be added (follow step 2 and 3). Remember to tell him he's doing a 'great job' or give other verbal praise for each element, such as reviewing the schedule, pointing to and verbalising the next activity, going to the area where the activity is to take place, and initiating the scheduled activity. Initially, he may need a prompt for each part of this chain.

Step 7. Initially, it may be necessary to provide extra motivation for completing the process (lots of praise, exaggerated high fives etc.) for specified elements of the described activity. This should be gradually faded and replaced with social praise as he becomes more independent in the process. When completely independent, social praise can be further reduced although not completely eliminated.

Step 8. As we know, daily schedules seldom remain unchanged during a day. Change happens all the time. The schedule will reduce the impact of change and help Josh better predict the course of the day. When a daily event is changed unexpectedly, a picture of the new activity should be substituted for the activity that will not be carried out and reviewed with Josh.

Step 9. The process of reviewing the schedule should be made increasingly longer. For example, reviewing might proceed according to the following schedule: (i) before every activity, (ii) before every two activities, (iii) in the morning, at noon, and before dinner, (iv) in the morning and at noon, and (v) in the morning. And more activities can be represented on each strip.

Step 10. If he refuses to participate in either checking his schedule or following through with an activity, simply state something like, 'I wonder what you are doing today? How can I find out? I know, I can look at your schedule book.' Pause, and give him a chance to join you. If he does not seem interested, say, 'Oh, I see first you are going to ______'. Describe the first activity. Then say, 'I wonder what comes after that'. Continue this process but do not force or overly prompt if he does not want to join in.

Other teaching methods

Other teaching methods include the following:

Personalised learning is an educational approach that aims to customise learning to each student's strengths, needs, skills and interests (Abawi, 2015). Each student gets a learning plan that's based on what they know and how they learn best. An example of this is an individualised education plan (IEP).

Intensive Interaction is an approach that focuses on interactions and aims to teach the fundamentals of communication. It was developed to promote early levels of communication development and it promotes 'conversation' through eye contact, facial expressions and vocalising (Caldwell, 2012). Nind & Hewett (1994) describe Intensive Interaction as both a way of teaching and a way of just being with a person. The focus is on developing an interaction style that matches the person you are supporting. Initially developed in a school in Harperbury, it was a method of learning (both for the person with intellectual disability and their support team). Nind & Hewett (1994) outline that the fundamentals of communication include:

- Using and understanding eye contact and facial expressions.
- Using and understanding sociable physical contacts.
- Using vocalisations with meaning (for some, speech development).
- Taking turns in exchanges of behaviour, and/or sequencing a social exchange with another person.
- Enjoying being with another person.

Conclusion

Person-centred planning and person-centred actions need to factor in people's lifelong learning aspirations and opportunities to sustain them. We need to focus on how we teach new skills rather than operate from the position that people cannot learn new skills. Having an interesting life, with interesting things to do alongside interesting people who value and support you, is a core component of having a good quality of life and an indicator of good support.

Person-centred planning methods are one way to capture people's aspirations, for example, person-centred active support creates opportunities to be engaged and have choice and control in what you do, when, and with whom. Positive behaviour support may help to identify the skills a person needs to learn to better meet

 Enabling Capable Environments © Pavilion Publishing and Media Ltd and its licensors 2024.

their own needs. Other approaches such as our capable environments appraisal or the Quality-of-Life appraisal are ways to identify opportunities and capture real, positive and quality outcomes for people with an intellectual disability, their families and those who support them.

Several teaching methods can be used to ensure you meet each person's needs when supporting them to develop their skills. You should focus on the person's preferences for what they want to learn, how they want to learn, and the pace at which they choose to learn. Remember, a good life and learning new skills must be planned for.

Enabling Capable Environments © Pavilion Publishing and Media Ltd and its licensors 2024.

Chapter 9: Person-Centred approaches to understanding behaviours that challenge

'When we use the person's perspective as a basis for ***understanding*** *why they act in the way they do, we are more likely to act in really helpful ways* ***with*** *the person rather than in strategies that work over or against the person.'*
(Lovett, 1996, p42)

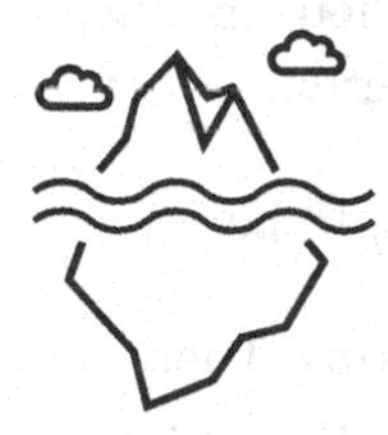

Chapter contents:

- Origins and current contemporary approaches to understanding behaviour.
- How contemporary approaches to assessment and understanding are informed by quality of life as part of interventions and outcomes.
- Quality of life and quality of supports inform person-centred approaches, such as positive behaviour support.
- An overview of functional assessment.
- Personalised supports that support a Comprehensive Functional Assessment.

Learning outcomes

After reading this chapter and completing the suggested activities and reflections, the reader should be able to:

- Discuss and identify the principles of understanding behaviours that challenge.
- Identify the barriers to quality-of-life outcomes in the context of assessment.

- Consider the process of Assessment, Planning, Implementation and Evaluation (APIE) in understanding behaviour that challenges and developing support based on this understanding.
- Understand behaviour and systems change.
- Appreciate the role of personalised and informed support.

Introduction

The quote at the beginning of this chapter reflects Herb Lovett's (1996) thoughts on the use of assessments and how their criteria are applied in practice. He reflects that tools that measure concepts such as a person's IQ, exam results and aptitude are at risk of being used to segregate and separate people; he draws similarities with how we define and quantify data about people's behaviour. For example, when assessment tools categorise behaviour as being attention seeking, or demand avoidance, we are stigmatising people and we therefore risk that people will respond to such categories of behaviour in a negative way and we fail to understand behaviour from the persons perspective.

Examples of negative responses might be:

- This behaviour is attention seeking. Therefore, we should ignore it.
- This behaviour is avoidant and, thus, this person must tolerate and accept the demand.
- This behaviour is because the person likes doing it. Therefore, they need to learn they cannot just do what they like when they like.

We would agree with Lovett's reflections and argue that such labels come from the perspective of the person conducting an assessment (fitting the person into the criteria of the assessment tool they are using) and can therefore lack real meaning or understanding of the person's perspective. Such negative linear conclusions from the assessment are biased and not person-centred. We are advocates of a more non-linear understanding of a person's behaviour in the context of what message the person is trying to convey and why, what their life experiences have been, and what their hopes and aspirations are, therefore leading to a more contextual understanding of why this behaviour is happening in the here and now. This leads us to consider the role of functional assessment in understanding why behaviours that challenge occur and to give the context of the circumstances within which they occur – moving away from seeing behaviours that challenge as something that need

 Enabling Capable Environments © Pavilion Publishing and Media Ltd and its licensors 2024.

to be managed, to understanding how we can better meet people's needs so such behaviour doesn't happen in the first place.

> 'Why would this person need to bang his head to get attention?" or even "Does he have so little control over his world that he needs to hurt himself or someone else to gain control?" In the context of a thorough functional analysis, such questions have helped us to use the behavioural technology in a more creative and humane manner. We exhort you to call upon your own creativity and skill in human interaction to do likewise.'
> (Donnellan *et al*., 1988)

Developing a functional understanding of behaviour was a pivotal change in how behaviours that challenge were understood and how people with an intellectual disability could receive better support. Having a functional understanding should lead to a functional support plan that better meets the person's needs. Developments in assessment tools led to new approaches and methods. The Questions About Behavioural Function (QABF) and Motivational Assessment Scale (MAS) were developed, meaning approaches such as experimental analysis were no longer needed. This was ethically correct, however, in some circumstances it led to a linear understanding that all behaviour was based on just four functions. We are sure that this was not the author's intent – they were trying to avoid the need for experimental analysis, which is commendable – but it did lead to (in some circumstances) a very singular and often misrepresented categorisation of behaviour, rather than a functional understanding. For example, this behaviour is attention seeking, this behaviour is demand avoidance (escape), this behaviour is… and so on. Such linear categorisation can lead to linear responses. This is not to say that these identified functions do not support our understanding of behaviour, but that there should be an acknowledgement of what this specifically means to the person within the context in which it occurs. Using tools which categorise behaviour typically miss this context.

The negative impact of this is that challenging behaviour is perceived as being predetermined and intentional, and therefore the person is in control of it. For example, if the function were to gain attention, some would argue that we should ignore it, so the person is not *'learning'* to seek attention. This is a dangerous assumption and leads to equally dangerous responses. For example, if a person is trying to make attempts to connect with you (gain your attention) and you ignore it, this can lead to an escalation of the behaviour and can lead to further isolation and segregation for the person. We would also question why would you think ignoring someone who is trying to interact with you be an appropriate response to anyone.

As a general principle, if you produce an assessment report or are provided with an assessment report that ends with a conclusion that the function of the behaviour is:

- Attention
- Sensory
- Tangible
- Escape

Then, upon receipt of such a report, you should thank the sender and ask for more information and clarity about the context and why this may be a function. Our point is that, while these categories are helpful to think about regarding potential functions of behaviour, they tell us nothing about the contextual meaning of someone's behaviour from the person's perspective and their life circumstances. Therefore, the assessment is incomplete and needs to be expanded.

Contextual meaning

> *'The meaning of behaviour emerges from its function in the larger system, not necessarily from the event itself.'* (Howell & Vetter, 1976)

We have referred to the phrase 'moving on from what's wrong with you to what's happened to you' (Johnstone *et al.*, 2018) in Chapter 11. The phrase is usually associated with understanding behaviour from a perspective of trauma and there is now a growing body of evidence that shows people with an intellectual disability are more likely to have experienced traumatic events (Beail *et al.*, 2021). Examples of this include:

- Being abused or victims of hate crime.
- Being subject to restraint or being over-medicated.
- Being isolated (not of their choosing).
- Losing their home and connections with loved ones, sometimes because of detention under the Mental Health Act. Many people are removed to a hospital setting with no clear plan to move back to a home of their own and of their choosing.

 Enabling Capable Environments © Pavilion Publishing and Media Ltd and its licensors 2024.

- Experience events that are referred to as complex trauma, for example, physical, emotional or sexual abuse.

More comprehensive research concludes that such traumatic events impact a person's emotional and physical well-being and should be considered in the context of understanding how a person may appear to be challenging. For example, Harding (2021) outlines several behaviours that can be associated with the experience of trauma, some of which can include aggressive or self-injurious behaviour, appearing disassociated or lacking interest in life. Without an understanding of the person's life history and the context of their current situation, the trauma experienced in a person's life could be missed, and there is a risk that teams could re-traumatise a person.

What needs to be considered in our attempts to support people is how our responses can, without necessarily intending it, be aversive or traumatising to the individual. This could risk making a situation worse as we don't have a contextual as well as a functional understanding of the behaviour that challenges.

Thinking space

Watch this short video (five minutes): 'Changing conversations: Understanding Behaviour – Raising Awareness of restrictive practices in the early years'. This is a resource from the Institute of Health Visitors, developed in collaboration with The Challenging Behaviour Foundation and The Sleep Charity.

https://vimeo.com/551420101/958680cc42

After watching, consider the following points:

- Think about how families are trying to navigate a way of understanding their child's needs.
- Consider how services that are meant to support the family are responding.
- Think about the trauma the child is experiencing, and the family members.
- What do you think the messages of the behaviour are and how do you believe people's responses help, or make the situation worse?

The purpose of this thinking space is to illustrate that it is very unlikely that a single assessment or screening tool would be able to identify the message of the behaviour in this scenario.

What is important is that the people around the person knew something was wrong and knowing and caring about the person helped them to work it out in a more collaborative and helpful way that was responsive to the child's needs.

We are not suggesting that assessments are not necessary – there is a wide range of evidence to show they are (NICE, 2015), but they must be used in the context of working collaboratively with the person and those who know them best (Gore et al., 2013; 2022).

Understanding behaviour

Multiple factors can influence our behaviour. However, research into many of these factors is still in its infancy, as is our understanding of how they affect behaviour. For example, a broader understanding of genetics, neurophysiological and psychological factors still need to be better understood (Bowring *et al.*, 2017; 2019). This means we continue to have a limited understanding of how and why behaviours that challenge occur. Expanding our understanding of these broader factors is essential if we are to understand how to better tailor and develop the support people need. While we await further developments, the most current evidence base is grounded in understanding the ecological and psychosocial variables, and the predominant area of current evidence-based practice comes in the form of positive behaviour support.

We use the terms 'challenging behaviour' or 'behaviour that challenges' as Jim Mansell in the RCP report (2007) states that:

'The phrase "challenging behaviour" is used in this report to include people whose behaviour presents a significant challenge to services, whatever the presumed cause of the problem…'

Mansell continues to clarify the origins of the term, saying:

'…When the term "challenging behaviour" was introduced, it was intended to emphasise that problems were often caused as much by the way in which a person was supported as by their own characteristics. In the ensuing years, there has been a

 Enabling Capable Environments © Pavilion Publishing and Media Ltd and its licensors 2024.

drift towards using it as a label for people. This is not appropriate, and the term is used in this report in the original sense.'

The term 'challenging behaviour' was coined by The Association for Severe Handicaps (TASH) in the USA in the late 1980s, with a view of focusing on the context in which challenging behaviours occurred, rather than labelling the individual as inherently 'challenging' (RCP, 2007). However, as Mansell points out, the term has drifted from understanding behaviours that challenge as being a social construct to the term becoming a diagnostic label that results in people with an intellectual disability being further marginalised as a result. What is needed is an understanding of what we mean by 'behaviours that challenge' to ensure people get access to the support and resources (including specialist input) in a timely way when it is needed.

Definitions of challenging behaviour

The most common definition of 'challenging behaviour' was first provided by Emerson in 1995 and again by Emerson & Enfield in 2011. In their work, they define challenging behaviour as:

'Culturally abnormal behaviour(s) of such an intensity, frequency, or duration that the physical safety of the person or others is likely to be placed in serious jeopardy, or behaviour which is likely to seriously limit use of, or result in the person being denied access to, ordinary community facilities' (Emerson, 1995; Emerson & Enfield, 2011).

The Royal College of Psychiatrists (2007) defined 'challenging behaviour' very similarly as:

'Behaviour of such an intensity, frequency, or duration as to threaten the quality of life and/or the physical safety of the individual or others and is likely to lead to responses that are restrictive, aversive or result in exclusion.'

We would suggest the definition of 'challenging behaviour' is updated to:

'Behaviours that challenge are of such severity, frequency or duration that they act as a barrier or threaten the person's quality of life and/or the physical and/or psychological safety of the individual or others and is likely to lead to responses that are restrictive, aversive or result in exclusion.'

Our updated definition makes three additional concepts more explicit in our understanding of behaviour that challenges.

The first is the inclusion of **severity (episodic severity)**, which recognises that how we define behaviours that challenge and the impact of this behaviour has progressed. We now understand better that simply thinking we need to make a behaviour stop is:

a. Limiting in an approach.
b. Not person-centred, for example, if we don't understand why the behaviour is happening and develop strategies which reflect this understanding, we are not addressing the person's support needs or the context of why this challenging behaviour occurs.
c. Fails to recognise the impact of the behaviour and how the reduction of its severity reflects the effectiveness of the plans Reducing the episodic severity of an episode of challenging behaviour is now considered evidence of effective personalised support planning.

There are specific ways to measure severity (episodic severity as outlined by LaVigna *et al*. (2022) and Spicer & Crates (2016)). More detail on episodic severity can be found in Chapter 11 but it is a variable factor that we now know is an indicator of the impact of challenging behaviour and a potential indicator of quality-of-life outcomes (see Chapter 1 for a wider discussion on quality of life). Ways to measure episodic severity can include severity scales, for example, for a behaviour that challenges such as damaging items, the scale might look like this:

- Level one: Throws a cup at the wall causing the cup to break (cup cost £1.50).
- Level two: Throws a cup and tea pot against the wall, marking the wall (cup cost £1.50 and paint to repair the wall cost £12.99).
- Level three: Throws the TV remote at the TV screen (TV screen repair £350).
- Level four: Pulls the top drawer of the dishwasher to the floor (cost to replace dishes £120 but also causes lacerations to feet when leaving the kitchen requiring first aid).

 Enabling Capable Environments © Pavilion Publishing and Media Ltd and its licensors 2024.

- Level five: Throws a bottle at someone's car (causing lacerations to the person's head requiring hospital treatment, and the cost to replace car glass is £500).

The importance of episodic severity scales is in their ability to help move away from 'we just need to "stop" or "manage" a behaviour', towards reducing the severity of each episode of behaviour that challenges. For example, if the severity is not reducing, this would suggest the person's plans need to be revised.

In summary, episodic severity is defined as a measurement of the gravity or seriousness of an episode of behaviour that challenges, and interventions should also be evaluated on their ability to reduce this severity (LaVigna *et al.*, 2022).

The second concept in our definition includes considering what acts as a **barrier to the person's quality of life**. When working with support teams, we often hear comments such as 'If only he would stop hitting people, we could go into the community' or, 'When he learns not to shout at people, we can go to the playground'. Here, opportunities to have a good life become are restricted by the person behaving or not behaving in a certain way, and their behaviour can become a barrier. Mansell (2007) stated that people need good support that meets their needs to have a good life irrespective of their behaviour. Please refer to Chapter 1 on ways to appraise quality of life.

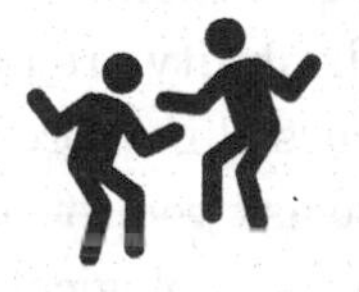

Our third addition to previous definitions of challenging behaviour is to include a risk to people's **psychological safety**, both in the context of the occurrence of behaviour and the responses to it.

Psychological safety means feeling safe to take interpersonal risks, to speak up, to disagree openly and to raise concerns without fear of negative repercussions.

Enabling Capable Environments © Pavilion Publishing and Media Ltd and its licensors 2024.

The term originated in research by Edmondson (1999; 2004) which considered the culture of workplace environments and concluded that workplace environments are more productive and effective when people feel psychosocially safe. From several studies (Aranzamendez *et al.*, 2015; Turner & Hander, 2018) we have summarised, in Figure 9.1 below, the core components of environments that reflect psychological safety.

Figure 9.1: Core components of psychological safety

A climate of open discussion
Creating opportunities for improvement
Willingness to learn
Feeling comfortable speaking up
Perception that you are accepted and valued
Trust
Not fearing recriminations
Ethical and reflective leadership
Benevolence and integrity

People with intellectual disability need to feel psychologically safe. Just as the people supporting them do – any compromise will result in people not feeling connected to the person they are meant to be supporting, leading to isolation for the individual. Without feeling psychologically safe, people with an intellectual disability can feel unsafe and fearful in their own homes; it creates a culture in which people with an intellectual disability are not valued or do not have any control over their lives. This is discussed in more detail in Chapter 1. In the context of rights and self-determination, we ask you to consider the support you provide and the impact this has on people's psychological well-being.

Enabling Capable Environments © Pavilion Publishing and Media Ltd and its licensors 2024.

Thinking space

'Behaviours that challenge are of such severity, frequency, or duration that they act as a barrier or threaten the person's quality of life and/or the physical and/or psychological safety of the individual or others and are likely to lead to responses that are restrictive, aversive or result in exclusion.'

Consider the following questions about this definition:

a. Does it help your understanding of what is meant by 'behaviour that challenges'?
b. Does it help your understanding of the impact of behaviour that challenges?
c. Does it prompt you to think about the person's quality of life?
d. Does it prompt you to think about how you respond to behaviour that challenges and is it helpful? For example, are your responses having a negative or positive impact on:
   - The person's quality of life?
   - The severity, frequency or duration of the behaviour?
   - The persons emotional and/or psychological well-being?

We would suggest that, if someone's behaviour does not fit within the above definition, it is likely not a behaviour that challenges and may be a misuse of the term that could lead to negative outcomes for the person such as exclusion or not being able to access the support they need.

What is positive behaviour support?

Positive behaviour support has several definitions, depending on how the definition is applied to different settings, such as a school setting or more generic settings, based on the country where the definition is applied. It may also depend on the context of the authors, for example, if they are from an academic or practice-based setting, or both. In this chapter, we will not align ourselves to one specific definition, but we will draw upon the common themes in each definition.

The term 'positive behaviour support' emerged in the 1980s out of the ethical dilemmas surrounding the use of what is considered aversive consequence- or punishment-based practices with people with intellectual disability (Johnston *et al.*, 2006). During this time, there was a growing recognition that more effective and ethical approaches, such as non-aversive strategies, should be implemented.

Positive behaviour support (PBS) is considered a framework based on person-centred values that include the science of applied behaviour analysis and use a data-driven approach to understanding why behaviours that challenge happen. It aims to teach individual skills and change the environment to meet a person's needs better (Gore *et al.*, 2013, 2022). The main aim of positive behaviour support is to increase the quality of life of the person and those around them, with behaviours that challenge being reduced as a side effect (Carr, 2002; Horner, 1990; LaVigna *et al.*, 2022). PBS involves understanding why challenging behaviours may occur, what increases the likelihood of behaviours that challenge, what maintains the challenging behaviour and the purpose or function it serves for the individual. It also considers the impact of the behaviour on the individual and those around them (Hastings *et al.*, 2013; Bowring *et al.*, 2017). There are many examples of PBS supporting effective and long-term change for people who display behaviours that challenge (LaVigna & Willis, 2012; McLaughlin *et al.*, 2012) and using this approach is considered best practice (NICE, 2015).

In summary, PBS encapsulates several core principles that focus on comprehensive lifestyle changes and quality of life, a life-span perspective, ecological validity, stakeholder participation, social validity, systems change and multi-component interventions, with an emphasis on prevention, flexibility with respect to scientific practices and multiple theoretical perspectives (Carr *et al.*, 2002).

Why is positive behaviour support needed?

Earlier in this chapter, we identified some of the limitations in how we understand behaviours that challenge. However, we currently have an array of knowledge from research that support the claim that the environment (the physical environment and the social environment) is an agent for setting the events for behaviours that challenge to occur or not occur.

For now, we will focus on these environmental factors to help us have a more contextual understanding of many of the variables that can act as setting events where behaviours that challenge occur or do not occur. In the context of positive behaviour support, this means that we consider all these variables in the context of the person's quality of life, physical and emotional well-being and the ability of service systems and processes to provide personalised support. All this information provides a broader context that addresses barriers to the person's quality of life and gives a more personalised context to the message that the behaviour that challenges may be communicating, as illustrated in Figure 9.2 below.

 Enabling Capable Environments © Pavilion Publishing and Media Ltd and its licensors 2024.

Figure 9.2: A contextual understanding of behaviours that challenge

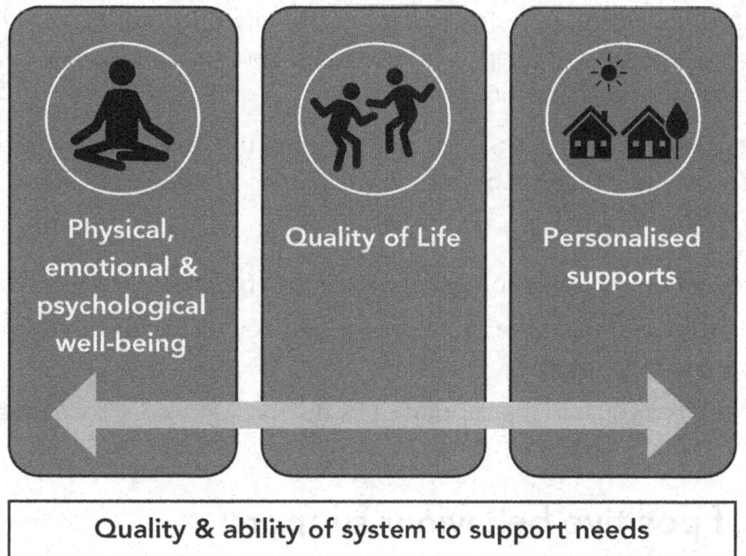

When approached from a comprehensive assessment perspective, this process can enhance our understanding of the person's quality of life and we avoid a linear perspective of what the problem behaviour is and how we 'fix/stop it'. Understanding from a quality-of-life perspective gives us a functional understanding of what the message is, but also a contextual understanding of why the message needs to be communicated.

We don't want to stop messages that convey:

- The person doesn't like something.
- The person is unhappy.
- Something isn't working for them.

We need to ensure that these messages are heard clearly and understood in a more deliberate way and that we listen and respond to those messages.

Enabling Capable Environments © Pavilion Publishing and Media Ltd and its licensors 2024.

Thinking space

Think about a time when you behaved in a way you are probably now quite embarrassed about. Perhaps you shouted at someone or threw something and stormed off angrily.

Spend a bit of time reflecting on that situation using the bullet points below and consider how each of these factors may have influenced how you behaved.

For example:

- How were you feeling, emotionally, physically and psychologically?
- How was your life at that time, were you missing key things in your life that make you happy and contented?
- Did you feel that you had the support of loved ones and work colleagues?

Process of positive behaviour support

Positive behaviour support involves a process of assessment (which can be brief or more detailed and comprehensive), but to reach a functional and contextual understanding it should include the four stages shown in Figure 9.3. These are:

- Assessment.
- Planning (detailed in Chapter 10).
- Implementation (detailed in chapters 6, 8 and 10).
- Evaluation (detailed in Chapter 5).

Figure 9.3: Process of positive behaviour support

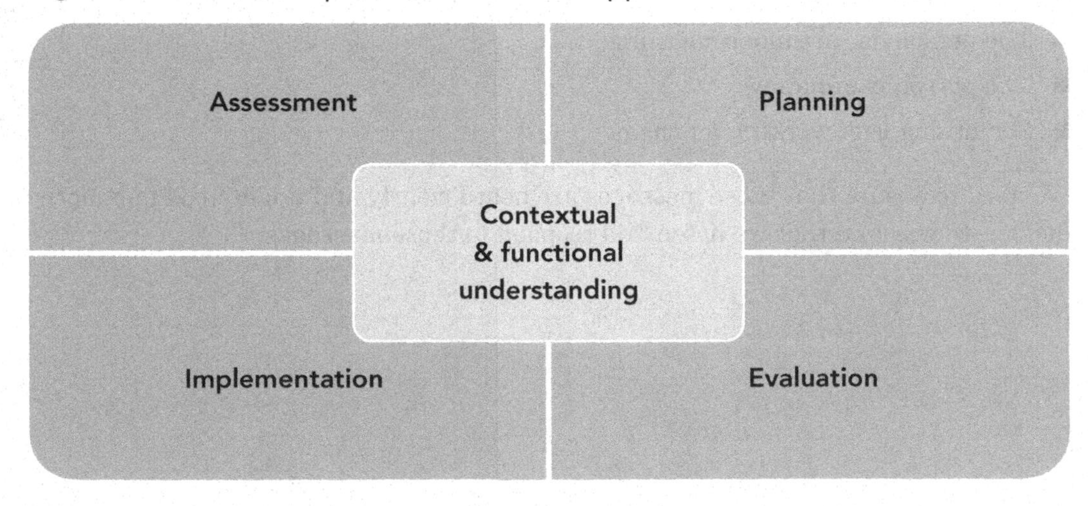

 Enabling Capable Environments © Pavilion Publishing and Media Ltd and its licensors 2024.

What are we trying to understand?

Assessment is the process of understanding what and why behaviours that challenge happen and then using that information to better meet the person's needs, and to enable those who support them to meet those needs. In summary, we are trying to understand the person's needs in the context of their quality of life and the quality and abilities of their support (Figure 9.4).

The most common format of assessment is referred to as a functional assessment, for which there are several tools that support a comprehensive functional assessment. These are detailed in Table 9.1 below.

Assessment

Figure 9.4: Assessment in positive behaviour support

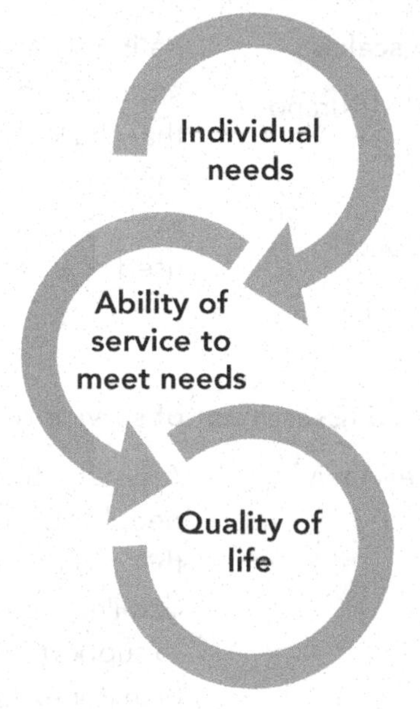

Table 9.1: Tools to support functional assessment	
Assessment tools which can support functional assessment	**Description**
Individual needs	
Physical well-being Health assessment, pain assessments, dementia screening and medication reviews (Emerson & Enfield, 2011; NICE, 2015).	Internal factors such as physical or mental health should be considered as contributing factors in the assessment and meaning of behaviours that challenge.
Mental health well-being Mini PAS-ADD & PAS-ADD, (Prosser *et al*, 1997; Moss *et al*, 1998).	Tools to help recognise the possible presence of a mental health need so that further referrals/investigations can occur.
Behaviours that challenge scales Motivation Assessment Scale (Durand & Crimmins, 1992). Questions about behavioural function (QABF; Matson & Vollmer, 1995) Measurement of Frequency, Duration and Severity (LaVigna *et al*, 2022).	Rating scales can provide a structured approach to understanding behaviours that challenge. Rating scales can suggest the potential function of the behaviour, but it is not recommended these are used in isolation.
Individual needs and assessment of service to meet those needs	
Functional assessment Interviews/ Questionnaires O'Neil, *et al* (2015).	A systematic approach to interviewing people about behaviours that challenge; this information can contribute to a more detailed formulation and understanding to support the development of a specific plan (for example a MEBS plan, see Chapter 10).
Observations ABCs, incident reports, other observation forms (Emerson & Enfield, 2011).	Direct observation in the person's natural setting, and considers the interplay of the immediate environment and those within the environment to help understand the contexts of why behaviours could be happening (and when they are not happening).

Enabling Capable Environments © Pavilion Publishing and Media Ltd and its licensors 2024.

Capable environments Appraisal Hume *et al* (2021), and in this book.	Appraisal of the quality of how support is organised and delivered.
Quality of life	
Active support measure Mansell *et al* (2005).	Can be used as a measure of quality of engagement and staff support.
Quality-of-life measures Family Quality of Life Scale (FQLS); Beach Centre on Disabilities (2006). Guernsey Community Participation and Leisure Assessment (GCPLA; Baker, 2021). Health of the Nation Outcome Scales – Learning Disability (HONOS-LD) (Roy, *et al*, 2002). The Maslow Assessment of Needs Scales – Learning and Intellectual Disabilities (MANS-LD) (Skirrow & Perry, 2009).	Can be used pre- and post-intervention to identify changes in quality of life. These can include overall quality of family life, improved community presence and participation. Where needed, improvements to overall health and well-being.
Other person-centred approaches (tools)	
Person-centred plans Department of Health (2012); NICE, (2015); O'Brien *et al* (2010). **Good lives model** Ward & Brown (2004).	Methods to develop individualised support through a planning process focused upon an individual's preferences and strengths.

People sometimes ask how many assessments you need to do, and the simple answer is that it's not about the number of assessments, it's about using what is needed to help you identify and better understand the person's needs and what must happen or change to better meet those needs. Therefore, an assessment may involve several of the tools above or there may just be a couple. However, best practice outlines that any assessment should include meeting with the person, spending time with them, and using data to inform decisions about what plans are needed and how the plan is working. Most of the assessment tools above can be accessed through health, social care or educational teams who have the relevant training and scope within their role to complete this and use the information to inform a positive behaviour support plan. We have listed many such assessments as an illustrative guide to what could be used, rather than being prescriptive. However, the most common assessment used in the context of developing a plan is a functional assessment, and we have therefore expanded our discussion to provide a guide to this type of assessment.

Functional assessment

Below, we will outline some of the typical steps that support the process of a functional assessment.

Step 1: Gathering information

It is important to gather as much information as possible about the person (this includes historical information). This can be done by speaking to the person, their family and friends, reviewing the person's support plan, other reports such as communication reports from a speech and language therapist, social worker reports, etc. There are several factors to consider when gathering information.

Speaking with the person and others in their life:

- Ensure you have consent to speak to people about the person and behaviours that challenge.
- Ensure that you are holding these meetings somewhere that is quiet, free of distractions and provides privacy. Make sure you have provided enough time to discuss topics in detail. This will allow open conversations and others won't feel pressured or restricted in what they can share. (See additional information later in this chapter about interviews.)
- Based on referral information or notes you may have taken from a review of records/documents, you are likely to have some questions to ask. A good place to start is to focus on what people would find helpful in the current situation, and to be aspirational about your role as being someone who can help improve things for everyone.
- Ask open-ended questions. Start your questions with 'what', 'why' and 'how'. This helps to gain detailed answers rather than simple yes or no responses.

 Enabling Capable Environments © Pavilion Publishing and Media Ltd and its licensors 2024.

- It is also important to allow the person you are speaking with to share information that isn't specific to your questions. You may gain great insights from this.
- With the above said, it is also important that the conversation stays focused on the individual and what is needed to best support them.
- Make sure you take notes from this discussion and clarify key points.

Reviewing records/reports:

- Ensure you have consent to access current and historical documents about the person.
- Make sure you gather a broad variety of information. Only taking information from one source could lead to the information being skewed to a specific period in that person's life or to a specific view of the individual and behaviours that challenge.
- At times, some reports can focus on behaviours that challenge and list these without the context or environmental factors that contributed to them. These reports can be focused on a problem rather than an understanding of the person's needs, so it is important to read them with an open mind and to try to understand the factors surrounding the behaviours that are described as challenging.
- You may come across historical behaviours that do not currently take place. It is important to be aware of these but not to allow them to influence decisions in the present, for example restrictions being applied without due cause.
- Make notes about how the behaviours that are described as challenging are described (i.e. what they look like).
- Make notes about key experiences or events that are significant to the person.
- Look at recommendations from previous reports. Were these recommendations actioned? If not, why not?
- What has worked well for the person in the past?

Step 2: Defining behaviour

Behaviours described as challenging must be defined in objective terms. This means describing what can be seen and what happens. This should not include why you think the behaviour that challenges are occurring or what the person could be feeling. Describing behaviour objectively increases the likelihood that everyone understands what the behaviour is that is causing a barrier to the person's quality

Enabling Capable Environments © Pavilion Publishing and Media Ltd and its licensors 2024.

of life or carries a risk for the person or others (see earlier discussion on the definition of challenging behaviour). It also means that the correct information about how often something happens, or how severe the impact is, is understood by everyone. If there are clear objective descriptions (i.e. what can be seen when the behaviour occurs), everyone can refer to them and identify whether this is what they saw happening. This will help to get more accurate data.

Identify the behaviour you want to define: This should be a behaviour that impacts the person's quality of life or that poses a risk to themselves or others. Some examples of impact could include the person being excluded from accessing spaces or events due to the behaviour that challenges. It may also be due to restrictions being placed on the person due to their or others safety, limiting their ability to learn new skills and access new experiences.

There may be several specific behaviours that occur together and can therefore be categorised together under a heading (i.e. shouting, banging doors or stamping feet being categorised as 'disrupting behaviour'). It is important to be cautious when categorising behaviours together as each individual behaviour may represent a different function or message.

Give the behaviour a short name: This can be helpful when there are a number of behaviours that are similar in how they present, and the short name provides a good summary of what is being seen (i.e. property destruction, physical aggression, verbal aggression, self-injurious behaviour, etc.).

When deciding on the short name, ensure that there is no intent implied by it. We do not know what the function/message of the behaviour is. That is what will be assessed during the functional assessment process. If we indicate the intent of the behaviour in the name we give it, we are unlikely to see behaviour objectively. It is likely to indicate a preconception of why the behaviour is occurring and this could influence other people's views of why the behaviour is occurring. The short name should:

- Convey the general category of the type of behaviour.
- Should be brief and should not indicate intent (i.e. do not use terms such as, angry behaviour, moody behaviour, not listening, ignoring, etc.).
- Not attempt to indicate why someone may be engaging in behaviours that challenge.

 Enabling Capable Environments © Pavilion Publishing and Media Ltd and its licensors 2024.

The short name should also be non-derogatory:

- We should not use terms which could be viewed negatively by others (i.e. manipulative, abusive, controlling).
- This could lead to others viewing behaviours that challenge negatively and treating the individual differently.

Provide a description of the behaviour that challenges: As well as a short name, you will also require a more detailed description of the behaviour. This is a description of what can be seen when the behaviours that challenge occur.

In summary

The behaviours that challenge should be defined objectively: This means we should only describe what we see/observe (i.e. what the behaviour looks like). The function or purpose should not be included in the description. We should define the behaviour based on what we can see when the behaviour occurs.

The definition should be clear: The definition should be specific and not open to interpretation. Two different people should be able to independently and accurately record whether the behaviour happened or not based on the description. It should be unambiguous.

The behavioural definition should have completeness: This might include a timeframe that indicates when one incident has finished and another has started. For example, an individual may engage in a behaviour that is described as challenging which is recorded as lasting 30 minutes, but it may be that in fact it lasted only two minutes, but restarted again a minute later, and this starting and stopping went on for 30 minutes. This clarity as to when a behaviour starts and stops is important because, if lacking, people will record a different number of incidents in the 30-minute timeframe – for example, some may record it as one event and others may record it as a higher number. The definition must be clear about when one incident has stopped and another has started.

Thinking space

Think about someone you support who has been described as engaging in behaviours that challenge. Think about what that behaviour looks like and try to define it.

Remember:

- Does the behaviour impact the person's quality of life or safety? Only then is deemed a behaviour that challenges.

Short name:

- General category.
- Brief.
- No intention indicated or implied.
- Non-derogatory.

Description of behaviour:

- Objective.
- Clear.
- Complete.

Step 3: Functional assessment interview

Current best practice guidance recommends that peer-reviewed assessment tools are used along with interviews with the person and those who support them, and the process also includes spending time with the person (direct observation). We outlined some of these in Table 9.1 above.

When completing an interview, ensure the environment is conducive to having confidential and possibly difficult conversations. Provide a quiet environment, free from distractions and interruptions, and make sure to have scheduled enough time to complete the interview comfortably. It is important when completing these assessment tools to ensure you do not allow any preconceived ideas about the function of a behaviour to influence you, the questions you ask or the person you are interviewing. Remember to ask open questions and allow interviewees time to speak and provide detail (i.e. use questions that start with, 'Tell me about…'). You may also use closed questions, which can give you a direct answer to a specific question (i.e. 'Does this happen during the school run?' 'What happens more,

 Enabling Capable Environments © Pavilion Publishing and Media Ltd and its licensors 2024.

property destruction or self-injurious behaviour?'). It is important to reflect back to the person what you think they have said and gain confirmation.

Observational assessments

Observations of behaviours that challenge are also key to assessing and identifying their function. It is preferable for observational assessments to take place in the person's usual environment and within their normal routines. This can be achieved through:

- Functional Assessment Observation Form (FAOF) (O'Neill *et al*, 2015).
- Time sampling.
- ABC charts.
- Scatterplots.

Before conducting observations, make sure everyone who is being observed knows why you are there and what the observation will entail. This is vital for everyone, including the focus person. You may need to consider different forms of communication that allow you to share this information with the focus person. It is important that any communication meets the person's preferred communication method. If those being observed are not aware of the purpose of the observations, they may rightly be upset or concerned.

Encourage those being observed to follow their usual routines and not to make changes due to your presence. If the focus person is visibly uncomfortable and this does not ease, or they want to speak to you and engage you in their activities, join in as this a great way to get to know the person. You may, however, need to consider another method for making observations, such as videoing routines and watching them later.

When your observation is concluded, wait until there is a natural stop in the activities that are taking place before explaining your observation is finished. Depending on the person, they may want you to sit for a while, engage in an activity or have a conversation. Make sure to say goodbye and let the person know when/if you will be back or when they may next see you.

Step 4: Interpretation

After gathering historical information, defining the behaviour and completing indirect assessments (interviews), and direct assessments (observations), it is now time to bring these together to help summarise the function of behaviour.

Enabling Capable Environments © Pavilion Publishing and Media Ltd and its licensors 2024.

Formulation and summary statements

Formulation is the process of pulling together the information gathered about the behaviour and the person, to develop a hypothesis as to the causes or functional relationship between variables and behaviours that challenge. This helps influence the strategies and interventions that are then used. The formulation should include:

- A clear and objective account of the behaviour that challenges.
- The variables (biological, medical, environmental – both physical or interpersonal) that influence (increase or decrease) and maintain the behaviour that challenges.
- A clear hypothesis (potential ideas) of the function/messages of behaviour.

There are several ways to summarise the findings from the assessment process. One is as a summary statement, for example.

Setting events	Antecedents	Behaviour	Consequence
These can be factors that make it more likely that behaviour that challenges could occur, for example some of the biological and environmental factors we discussed earlier in this chapter.	Factors that happen more immediately before the behaviour occurs that are closely linked to what the message of the behaviour is, for example, some demand is made or the person being in a situation they are finding difficult etc.	The clearly defined behaviour.	Factors that happen after the behaviour that could contribute to the behaviour happening again. Factors that resolve the situation quickly. Factors that make the situation worse.

Another way to present information from the assessment is as a formulation, one example is using the 5 Ps (Johnstone *et al.*, 2006)

Enabling Capable Environments © Pavilion Publishing and Media Ltd and its licensors 2024.

What is the **presenting problem**? The clearly defined behaviour	What are the **predisposing factors**? Consider all factors throughout the person's lifetime that could have contributed to the development of the problem.	What are the **precipitating factors**? What has worsened/ triggered the problem?	What are the **perpetuating factors**? What internal and external factors play a role in maintaining this situation.	What are the **protective factors**? Describe strengths and qualities of the person that can help.

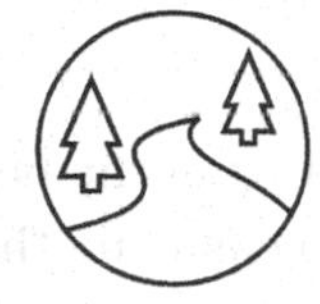

Pathways to success

- Be clear in any descriptions of behaviour that challenges. Consider how it maps to our definition of behaviours that challenge. If it doesn't, then you need to question why the behaviour is being considered as challenging.
- Be clear as to what is contributing to the person's quality of life and what is creating barriers to their achieving this.
- A positive behaviour support plan should not be used to fix deficient environments, for example if it is known that the person is living somewhere unsuitable, this should be addressed; if the person does not have the support they need, then this should be addressed.
- A positive behaviour support plan should contain detailed information about how to create a more capable environment that better meets the person's needs.
- Use data to inform what you are doing and why, but be mindful of capturing data that reflects positive aspects of someone's life – people are more than a data point on a graph.

Enabling Capable Environments © Pavilion Publishing and Media Ltd and its licensors 2024.

- Keep a focus on quality of life and what systems of support are needed to support it.
- Positive behaviour support assessment and plans are evolving and dynamic, and they should be aspirational. People are more than a collection of problems for professionals to 'fix'.
- Co-production is integral – it is not something that happens after the fact, we don't produce an assessment or a positive behaviour support plan and ask people what they think. The person, their families and their support teams are vital to ensuring an evidence-based assessment is made which informs practice and support.
- Use specialist support and input as needed.
- Formulations can improve our understanding of behaviours that challenge, allowing for a deeper understanding of 'what happened' rather than asking 'what is wrong with them?' when reflecting on incidents with clients.

Conclusion

Understanding behaviour in the context of the person's quality of life and their systems of support is fundamental to ensuring the focus stays on what the person needs and how the system of support around them can provide this. So, why do we need a process of assessment? Many of us can work out why a person we live with behaves in a particular way, and most of the time we respond in helpful ways. But this understanding is based on long-term relationships and a wish for wellness for the person we love. This emotional and relational connection is almost conditioned out of us as professionals (see Chapter 1) and we can miss key determinates of the person's quality of life and self-determination. Hence the need to ensure the person's loved ones are central in assessment and planning.

Enabling Capable Environments © Pavilion Publishing and Media Ltd and its licensors 2024.

Chapter 10: Development of multi-element behaviour support plans

'Science tells us how we can change things, but values tell us what is worth changing.'
(Carr, 1996)

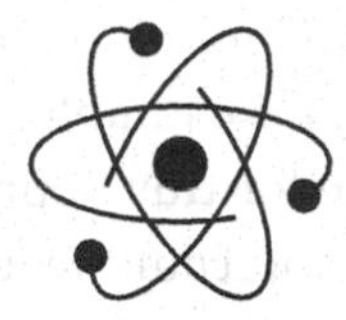

Chapter contents:

- What is Multi-Element Behaviour Support (MEBS)?
- The components of a MEBS plan?
- Person-focused training.
- Implementing a MEBS plan.
- Monitoring a MEBS plan.
- Pathways to success.
- Discussion questions.
- Conclusion.

Learning outcomes

After reading this chapter and completing the suggested activities and reflection, the reader should be able to:

- Understand how a MEBS plan is developed.
- Identify the components and elements of a MEBS plan.
- Determine the links between a functional understanding of behaviour and the MEBS plan.

- Apply the principles of person-focused training.
- Establish methods to implement and support a MEBS plan.

Introduction

The quote by Carr (1996) at the top of this chapter should serve as a reminder that, whatever role we are in, the person we are supporting should remain central to what we are doing and why we are doing it. We should focus on whether what we do is of value to the person and is important to them. Research in the late 1980s began to identify the functional and communication elements of behaviour that challenges that we need to consider. At this time, many support approaches still focused on the individual and what was perceived as their problem behaviour, and many components of these approaches that were implemented to support the person were based on contingency management, for example, reinforcement. While research at that time did provide some evidence for this approach, it was identified that such a singular approach was insufficient and could lead to aversive approaches that were not valued by the individual or those supporting them.

Understanding how and why behaviours that challenge may or may not occur led to more functional and contextual support planning (discussed in detail in Chapter 9). By early 2000, as advances in research and policy developed, the role of support systems and the environment began to inform a more non-linear (multi-component) approach to how support for people with an intellectual disability should be organised and provided. This shift in thinking included more ethical and person-focused approaches that are valuable to the person.

As a core principle, it is now recognised that plans to support behaviour practices of teams/supports are only valid if they have an impact on:

- Increasing the person's quality of life (increasing choice, control, opportunities, meaningful relationships and community access).
- Enhancing skills and opportunities, focused on quality-of-life goals and outcomes.
- The enabling of personalised supports and environments, which in turn bring about a reduction of behaviours that challenge.
- A comprehensive understanding of the person's needs, and this understanding should include evidence-based approaches to assessment.

 Enabling Capable Environments © Pavilion Publishing and Media Ltd and its licensors 2024.

The research of early 2000 began to recognise that behaviour supports needed to be comprehensive and multi-component to ensure all the variables which contribute to the likelihood of challenging behaviour occurring were addressed, but more importantly, that positive behaviour support plans enhanced people's quality of life.

What is a multi-element behaviour support plan?

In 2005, LaVigna & Willis developed the multi-elemental support plan which provided the comprehensive features of assessment and multi-element behaviour support plans (MEBS). When outlining the MEBS model, LaVigna & Willis stress that the focus of research and application in PBS may have relied on individual interventions, leading to a misunderstanding of PBS as a standalone intervention that disregards the broader context and outcomes. The consequence of this is that professionals may incorrectly use standalone strategies aimed at addressing a specific concern. The result is that these strategies may not take into consideration a person's whole life, leading to temporary changes in small areas but no broad and long-standing quality-of-life outcomes. They propose that the integrated MEBS model, involving a focus on several interventions and a holistic approach to address all aspects of a person's life, is required to fully understand and support change, with a particular focus on outcomes related to quality of life, choice, independence, relationships and engagement.

This multi-element behaviour support plan is based on a comprehensive functional assessment (see Chapter 9) and considers the system of support around the individual. It is orientated in a constructive and educational approach where interventions and supports are focused on what is being added to lead to improvements in a person's quality of life.

Later, Doody (2009) showed that multi-element behaviour support is a structured model that supports the delivery of PBS in the context of a person's human rights as it focuses on increasing quality of life and engagement, through enhancing a person's independence and skills, and, critically, changing the environment to better meet the person's needs. MEBS incorporates a range of proactive and reactive strategies that consider a person's whole life, and together, these strategies increase quality of life and decrease the likelihood of future behaviours that challenge (McClean & Grey, 2012a; 2012b).

Enabling Capable Environments © Pavilion Publishing and Media Ltd and its licensors 2024.

Table 10.1: Overview of multi-element behaviour support plans

Proactive			Reactive
Environmental strategies	**New skills and opportunities**	**Prevention strategies**	**Resolution (reactive) strategies**
■ Physical environment. ■ Interpersonal environment. ■ Programmatic environment. ■ Philosophy and values.	■ Fun skills. ■ General skills. ■ Functional skills. ■ Equivalent replacement skills. ■ Coping skills.	■ Managing antecedents. ■ Increasing preferred events (including people). ■ Differential schedules of reinforcement.	■ Non-functionally based. ■ Functionally based.

(Adapted and updated from LaVigna *et al.*, 2022)

A multi-element behaviour support plan aims to include all the elements necessary for supporting people whose behaviours that challenge are a barrier to a good quality of life. It is based on a comprehensive and functional understanding of all the variables needed to enhance the person's quality of life. It reduces the variables that contribute to when and why behaviours that challenge occur.

The components of a multi-element behaviour support plan

Four elements in the MEBS plan fit under two overarching components, proactive and reactive support (see Table 10.1). We will summarise these two components next, and then explore each of them in more detail.

Proactive strategies

The first component is **proactive strategies**. These strategies aim to align the systems and supports to enhance a person's quality of life by personalising supports that fulfil their wants and preferences and that address the functional relationships between behaviours that challenge and the person's needs. Given this quality of life and personalised support focus, these plans are long-term strategies, and they

Enabling Capable Environments © Pavilion Publishing and Media Ltd and its licensors 2024.

should be dynamic, evolving and developing as the person's needs and wishes develop.

The elements of proactive strategies are:

- **Environmental/ecological strategies**, which aim to organise the person's support to meet their needs by understanding the variables that contribute to their overall well-being and quality of life. They also address the variables contributing to behaviours that challenge, such as the setting events identified in the functional assessment.
- **New skills and opportunities** aim to help the person achieve life opportunities and goals. It also teaches them skills to enhance their quality of life and to enable them to communicate or meet their needs, having identified the functional relationship between the person's behaviour and the skills that may be of value to them.
- **Preventative strategies** aim to reduce or avoid the known circumstances (from the assessment) to decrease the likelihood of behaviours that challenge occurring.

Resolution strategies

The second overarching component is **resolution strategies**, which aim to provide clear plans for responding when challenging behaviour occurs.

Resolution strategies are designed to respond to incidents safely and rapidly when they occur. These strategies are focused on something other than teaching (which occurs in the proactive part of the plan). These strategies are focused on situational management where the emphasis is on reducing the episodic severity of incidents. These resolution strategies include:

- Non-function-based reactive strategies in cases where we do not understand why the behaviour is happening.
- Function-based-reactive strategies in cases where we understand why this behaviour is occurring.

Both approaches are non-aversive and are marked in that they are designed to resolve a situation, prevent further escalation, and reduce the episodic severity of the incident with dignity and respect for the person (detailed in Chapter 11).

Enabling Capable Environments © Pavilion Publishing and Media Ltd and its licensors 2024.

Environmental/ecological strategies

Let us look now in more detail at environmental/ecological strategies. These strategies are essential to creating a contextual fit between the individual and their environment. By contextual, we mean everything in the environment is aligned to meet the person's individual needs. This part of the plan therefore helps to address the mismatch between the environment and the person's needs.

Table 10.2: Overview of environmental strategies
Physical environment: ■ Predictable support which honours the person's preferences*. ■ Sensory needs and preferences – acceptable physical environment*. ■ Opportunities for choice and control*. **Interpersonal environment:** ■ Considers attachment and attunement. ■ Relationships with friends and family*. ■ Positive social interactions, which focus on staff rapport and support style. ■ Communication strategies that consider the person's abilities and preferences. ■ Opportunities to learn new skills which are *fun* and *fun*ctional to the person. **Service environment:** ■ Variety of interesting people and activities. ■ Support staff are skilled in the personalised support the person needs*. ■ Staff are trained and skilled in the methods of communication the person needs and prefers. ■ Consistent and predictable routines and supports. ■ Health promotion and support. ■ Teams are supported, and reflective supervision and coaching provide practice leadership.

Enabling Capable Environments © Pavilion Publishing and Media Ltd and its licensors 2024.

Philosophy and values within the environment:

- People in the setting value the person and personalise their support.
- Staff are reflective, mindful, and skilled in personalised supports*.
- External involvement is routine in the support from families, advocates and those who are important to the person. There is a routine level of accountability and monitoring driven by the individual and those important to them.

*Many of these elements are discussed in more detail in chapters 2 to 4.

By making these changes to the environment, we aim to enhance the opportunities for the person to lead a fulfilling life, and we can also address the setting events and contexts where behaviours that challenge are more likely to occur. When informed by a functional assessment, the latter is only achieved by clearly understanding the function of the person's behaviour.

Teaching skills and enabling opportunities

This category focuses on enhancing skills and creating opportunities for the person to increase their independence, support access to new experiences, and increase their self-esteem. It also identifies the skills the person may need to indicate things are not working for them. In Chapter 7, we established that behaviours that challenge could serve a function or as a message to be understood. Based on this premise, we therefore need to consider what skills can replace the challenging behaviour to ensure needs are being met.

For example, does the person need a way to communicate that they do not like something and want it to stop or engage in activities that are not dangerous to themselves or others? For example, learning to discriminate between edible and non-edible items.

Table 10.3: Overview of teaching skills and developing opportunities

(See also Chapters 7 and 8)

Fun skills:

- Skills that the person wants to learn and develop.
- These skills may begin with a person-centred active support approach in which the focus is on trying things out and experiencing new opportunities.

General and functional skills:

- Increasing independence through teaching day-to-day skills (i.e. cooking, self-care, shopping, etc.) and skills linked to what the person enjoys doing (i.e. putting on their favourite music, shows, learning to play an instrument, etc.)

Functional equivalent skills:

- These are skills that are taught because they meet the same function as the behaviour that challenges but which better communicate or meet the person's need:
  - I am confused I don't understand what you are asking of me.
  - This task is too hard.
  - I am scared/lonely.
  - The noise is hurting my head.
  - I need a drink/something to eat.
  - I need it to be quieter.

Functionally Related Skills:

- These are skills that are related to the function/message of the behaviour, so while they do not replace the message directly, they relate to it.
- For example, if someone finds it difficult moving from one activity to another, teaching them how to use a now and next board can address the anxiety of the situation.

Coping skills:

- These could be situations that the person cannot easily remove from their life or are linked to preferred events that the person wants to access, such as waiting for buses or taxis, managing busy environments to access enjoyable activities (live sporting events, concerts, etc.), accepting feedback to progress in learning a new skill (playing an instrument, using specific tools, driving a car), etc.

Enabling Capable Environments © Pavilion Publishing and Media Ltd and its licensors 2024.

Prevention/focused support strategies

Prevention strategies are used in two ways. First, they serve as a short-term plan to avoid situations where we know, through assessment, that behaviours that challenge may occur. These are short-term strategies, while the strategies in the environment and skills teaching section take time to develop. For example, if we know that being in a busy supermarket is going to lead to behaviours that challenge, then, as a short-term plan while we are working out why (making an assessment), we might recommend the person avoids going to the supermarket, and shops online instead.

The second role they play is the prevention of escalation, for example, if we know that a person will shout before they throw an item at the wall, we don't wait for the person to throw the item, we might redirect them when they shout to their favourite songs on their iPad.

Some of these strategies may seem counterintuitive, but if we think in terms of the wider MEBS plan and of the bigger picture, which is to prevent a situation from escalating and ensure the environment is set up to work for the person in the context of their quality of life, then they make sense.

Table 10.4: Overview of prevention strategies
Prevention/focused support strategies
Managing antecedents: ■ These are factors that are known to increase the likelihood of challenging behaviour, sometimes referred to as setting events – therefore things we need to avoid doing. ■ Examples of this include not presenting requests in a demanding way, and avoiding certain situations, words or people. Increasing preferred events (including people): ■ These are factors which are known to be associated with a reduced likelihood of challenging behaviour occurring – therefore things we will do more of or that the person should have access to all the time. ■ Examples of this might be activities the person likes to do, places the person likes to be, more time with people they like, and free access to preferred items, for example their iPad.

Enabling Capable Environments © Pavilion Publishing and Media Ltd and its licensors 2024.

Differential schedules of reinforcement:

- Can and should only be used as a short-term strategy while a more detailed assessment is being undertaken along with making changes to the environment/skills teaching strategies. For example, encouraging/reinforcing the use of a sensory chew band instead of biting; note that this is a short-term strategy to reduce the likelihood of someone biting while the assessment is trying to understand the function and address this in a proactive way.
- If the function is assessed as providing a positive sensory need, this may be continued longer-term, but if the function is identified as a way of telling someone to leave, for example, the band may not be required and the person may be supported to communicate to others to leave their space.

Resolution strategies

> *'The role of a reactive strategy is to keep people safe in the here and now; not with an intent to influence change in the future.'*
> (LaVigna & Willis, 2005)

The use of resolution strategies is discussed in detail in Chapter 11.

The term 'NARS' was first outlined in the work of Crates & Spicer (2016) and Spicer & Crates (2016). It stands for non-aversive reactive strategies. In their work, they summarise NARS as being a way to respond to behaviour challenges or crises which do not involve the use of punishment or ways that the person would find aversive, for example the use of restrictive practices.

They outline two categories of NARS, the first being function-based NARS, where the function of behaviour has been assessed and understood. The second is non-function-based NARS, where the reason for the behaviour is not understood.

Remember, a reactive strategy aims to keep people safe in the here and now, and this is typically best done by responding to what the person needs.

Enabling Capable Environments © Pavilion Publishing and Media Ltd and its licensors 2024.

Table 10.5: Overview of non-aversive reactive strategies
Non-aversive reactive strategies (more detail in Chapter 11)
■ Redirection. This could involve redirecting the person to something you know the person likes or finds calming, a walk in the garden, a reminder of an event that is coming up, or asking them to help you with something you know they like to do. ■ Stimulus change. This involves bringing a new stimulus into the environment (i.e., introducing music into the room, etc.). ■ Active listening. The key to active listening is reflecting the emotions and messages that appear to be being communicated by the person, for example I see you are upset, this is hard, isn't it?

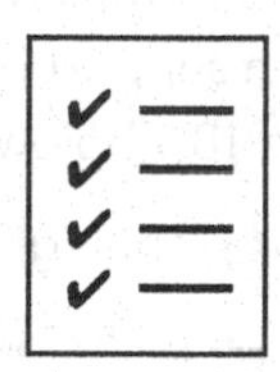

Benefits of MEBS

There are several key outcomes from the MEBS model and the impact it can have on the person. These are summarised as follows:

Quantitative improvements, which include:

- Increases in functional skills and opportunities.
- Reductions in the frequency of behaviours that challenge over time.
- A more immediate reduction in the episodic severity of the behaviour (LaVigna & Willis, 2005).
- Increasing access to less restrictive settings.
- The maintenance of these measures over time.

Qualitative improvements, which include:

- The reduction of barriers to success in the person's life.
- The person's needs are met.
- Higher density of activities that the person finds enjoyable occurring in all parts of the day.

Enabling Capable Environments © Pavilion Publishing and Media Ltd and its licensors 2024.

- Using learned skills across different settings.
- More choices about all aspects of life, independence, etc.
- An increased understanding by those involved with the person as to who the person is as a person, rather than focusing exclusively on behaviours that challenge.
- An increase in upholding peoples human rights.

(Hughes *et al*., 2014; Hume et al., 2021; LaVigna & Willis, 1996; Doody, 2009)

Thinking space

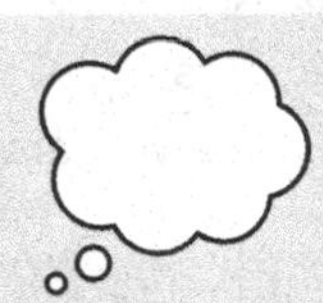

We acknowledge there are multiple formats for positive behaviour support plans, and we present just one format (MEBS). However, we would consider that all formats of such support plans should include, at a minimum, the principles in Figure 10.1 below.

Using Figure 10.1: Principle of support planning, consider the following points:

- Do you have plans which encompass the following principles?
- Do you have training in understanding and applying these principles?
- Are these principles discussed as part of the team's meetings/supervision/review meetings?
- What are the gaps in your support plans and what help is needed to address them?

 Enabling Capable Environments © Pavilion Publishing and Media Ltd and its licensors 2024.

Figure 10.1: Principles of support planning

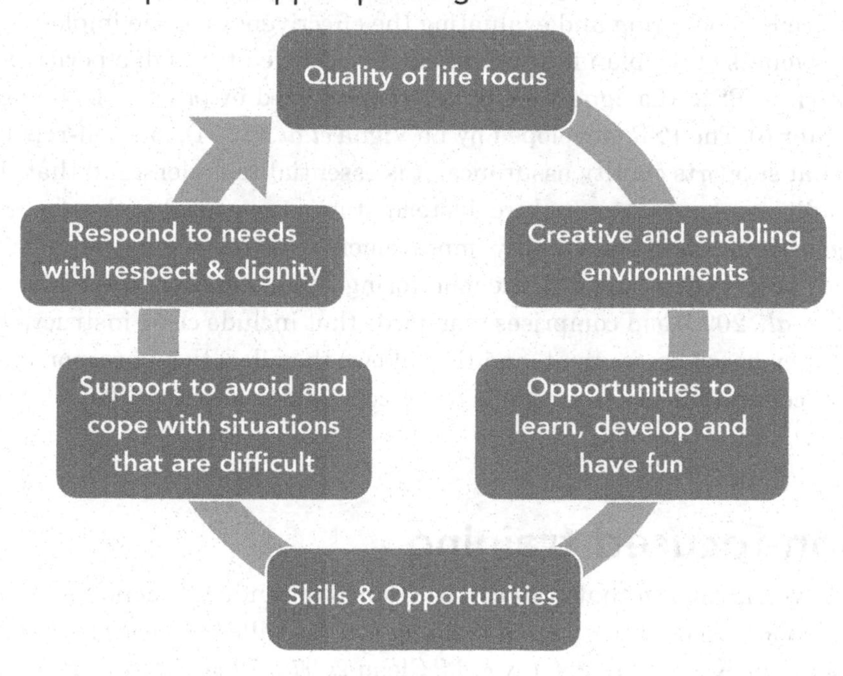

All strategies within the MEBS plans are based on an understanding of the function of behaviour, identified through a functional assessment (LaVigna & Willis 2005; LaVigna *et al.*, 2022). As well as a functional assessment, it is important that a MEBS plan is informed by the individual's background and history. Particular attention should be placed on the person's rights, needs and wishes, and that the strategies have an overall focus on the person's quality of life. This should also include their preferred communication methods, sensory needs, health factors, their motivations, and their environment (Doody, 2009). Other person-centred approaches, such as person-centred planning and quality-of-life domains should inform the development of the plan (more detail on these approaches is found in Chapter 1).

In addition to the assessment of the function and context of behaviours that challenge and the development of the MEBS plan, there is also a requirement to support those who implement the plan in practice. This includes teaching them the skills needed to support the person as well as teaching the enhanced skills that are required to implement the MEBS plan. Specific training in understanding how a MEBS plan is developed and the training and resources to implement and evaluate this will be required.

As a MEBS plan is a dynamic plan that evolves and changes according to the person's needs, monitoring and evaluating the effectiveness of the implementation and effectiveness of the plan is key. This can be achieved through a periodic service review (PSR) (Lavigna &Willis, 2005) supported by practice leadership (see Chapter 6). The PSR, developed by La Vigna *et al.* (1994), is a self-reporting process that supports quality assurance. It is essential to understand that this is not an audit or inspection procedure; instead, it is an appraisal with a focus on fully engaging in continuous quality improvement. It is a behaviourally-derived, structured process that supports the monitoring and evaluation of the MEBS plan (Lavigna *et al*., 2022) and comprises standards that include clear instructions and a competency-based assessment, and that allows the allocation of responsibility to ensure procedural fidelity (the plan is being completed as stated). This is detailed in Chapter 5.

Person-focused training

Studies have also shown that staff can be trained to conduct functional assessments and develop MEBS plans through a training process called person-focused training (PFT) (McClean & Grey 2012; Grey & McClean 2007; McClean *et al*., 2005). In fact, McClean *et al.* (2005) make the argument for training staff for to two key reasons:

1. There are a limited number of behavioural specialists/psychologists who can provide this vital support to individuals and their teams, leaving many without essential provision.
2. The better contextual fit (the fit between behavioural plans and the factors that affect implementation in a setting), the higher the chance plans will be implemented and maintained over time.

Staff who work with the person have a better understanding of the person and are acutely aware of the environmental and organisational factors that could hinder or enhance the implementation and maintenance of MEBS plans making them better placed to make decisions.

In 2005, McClean *et al*, developed and delivered a training programme called person-focused training (PFT) to staff working with individuals who engage in behaviours that challenge. The programme involved training staff to develop an understanding of the function of behaviour for an individual and then develop, implement and evaluate the effectiveness of a multi-element behaviour support plan. Staff developed plans that addressed changes to the environment, learning

 Enabling Capable Environments © Pavilion Publishing and Media Ltd and its licensors 2024.

skills, direct intervention (differential reinforcement, increasing preferred events, etc.), and reactive strategies. Vital to the implementation was the introduction of the PSR based on the recommendations from the assessment and subsequent support plan. McClean *et al* (2005) found:

- A 77% reduction in behaviours that challenge.
- Reductions in behaviours perceived as challenging were maintained at a 22-month follow-up.
- MEBS plans could be developed and implemented by direct support staff and frontline managers. These plans were found to be as effective as those plans that were designed by specialists.

This study was replicated in 2007 by Grey & McClean, which found:

- Approximately 66% of participants' behaviour that was perceived as challenging fell below 30% of baseline levels.
- Approximately 33% of participants had a reduction of between 30% and 70% of baseline levels.
- Training staff in developing and delivering MEBS plans was effective in reducing behaviours that challenge.

McClean & Grey (2012a) also researched the implementation of PFT with frontline staff over nine months:

- They found a reduction in behaviours that challenge for approximately 80% of people identified as a focus person within the programme, emphasising the acceptability and effectiveness of training frontline staff in the assessment, development, implementation and evaluation of MEBS.
- In their analysis, the authors identified that one factor had a significant influence on the reduction in behaviour and this was the acceptability of the intervention to the team. The authors also found high acceptability of the interventions being implemented.
- Lastly, and strikingly, they also found that no single intervention or type of intervention being implemented was linked to a decrease in behaviours that challenged. They suggest this further highlights the importance of the multi-elemental nature of PBS.

Enabling Capable Environments © Pavilion Publishing and Media Ltd and its licensors 2024.

Vital elements of PFT

There are several key elements to delivering and embedding PFT:

- Classroom-based training is an important part of the programme and allows the sharing of knowledge and theory between the trainer and participants.
- Critical to this is the application of evidence-based theory, and turning it into practical skills with the use of in-service coaching and mentoring. After more formal learning takes place, the trainer or someone in a specialist/leadership role spends time with the participants to practice the skills taught and feedback is provided to apply these new skills.
- System supports need to be in place to ensure these skills are maintained over time. Examples of this might be the use of progress meetings, supervision and an appraisal process (McClean *et al*., 2005).

Case study

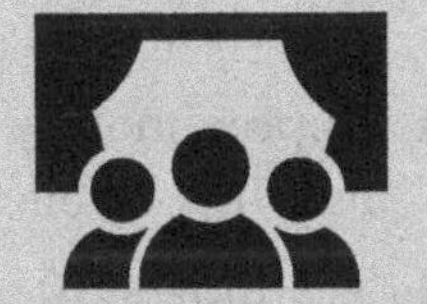

Below, we will detail how MEBS plans have been developed and implemented by frontline managers to increase quality of life and reduce behaviours that challenge. Throughout this case study, we will also provide useful resources that will allow the reader to replicate this process and facilitate MEBS within their own home, classroom or service.

Implementing a MEBS plan

The MEBS model was a key consideration in the work conducted by Hume *et al*. (2021). The model was used to train frontline managers to assess the function of behaviour that challenged and implement and evaluate MEBS plans.

Each frontline manager had selected a focus person with whom they had completed previous work as part of the pilot programme (see Chapter 2). In line with the capable environment's framework, this could be sufficient, for most people, and provide the support required to increase the focus person's quality of life and, as a side effect, reduce behaviours that challenge. For those managers who had not seen the significant impact on quality of life and behaviours that challenge, there was a requirement for additional training and support. These managers were asked to conduct a functional assessment to identify the function of challenging behaviour that the person would regularly engage in.

Enabling Capable Environments © Pavilion Publishing and Media Ltd and its licensors 2024.

With support from the trainers, the frontline managers were asked to:

- Gather historical information about the person by speaking to those who knew the person well.
- Define, with support, the behaviour that challenged using objective language.
- Interview the person's staff team and the person's friends and family, using peer-reviewed assessment tools, and discuss the behaviours that challenge.
- Complete observations of the focus person in their day-to-day activities and interactions.

This process helped the trainers to understand the contingencies surrounding the behaviour. This data was drawn together in a short assessment report which identified the function of behaviour that challenged, the motivating operations (setting events), antecedents and consequences.

The managers were then supported to use the functional assessment to develop a MEBS plan. Please see Chapter 9 for more information on how to conduct a functional assessment.

After hypothesising the function of the behaviour(s) that challenges, it is important to ensure this assessment influences the interventions implemented. In their pilot programme, Hume, *et al*. (2021) provided support and training to frontline managers to develop and implement a MEBS plan for each focus person, based on the completed functional assessment. Each frontline manager was supported to consider multiple strategies that would be implemented within each section of the MEBS plan. Managers were asked to review the information they had gathered as well as speak to stakeholders about the plans they felt were most important to the focus person's quality of life and well-being.

A reminder from Chapter 9 of what we mean by functions and messages of challenging behaviour is in Table 10.6 below. Remember behaviour may have more than one function.

Table 10.6: Summary of functions and messages of behaviour	
Function of behaviour (general category)	Message of behaviour (specific and personalised message of need)
Tangible	I need to get... I need to keep this close it helps me/I like it/I don't want to lose it.... I don't know when I can have it again.
Attention	Don't forget about me. I like being with you. Can you help me. I need to know what is happening next.
Sensory	I need to do this. I don't have any other way to do this. I like how this feels/smells.
Escape	I can't do this. This is scary. I feel dizzy just thinking about it. I don't understand. This is too much. I don't like how you are speaking to me.

Developing a MEBS plan

To create a MEBS plan, strategies must be developed within each element of the model. Multiple strategies/plans within each area will be important in ensuring a holistic approach to increasing quality of life and decreasing behaviours that challenge. Decisions about what plans to implement should be based on the information gathered during the functional assessment. Look back at Table 10.1 and remember all the areas that need to be considered when developing a MEBS plan.

 Enabling Capable Environments © Pavilion Publishing and Media Ltd and its licensors 2024.

Environmental strategies

Reviewing the information gathered will help in selecting the right environmental (ecological) strategies. Consider the summary statements in Table 10.6 above (and see Chapter 9), in particular the motivating operations/setting events along with the historical information, and identify if any clear 'triggers' continue to be raised. Review the information from your discussions with the person – did they discuss specific environmental factors that they like/don't like? Don't forget any other tools such as a person-centred plan, a sensory and/or health assessments.

When considering the information you have gathered, ask yourself:

- Does the environment meet the person's sensory needs?
- Is the person's home warm and welcoming?
- Is the environment organised in a way that the person can access what they want and need?
- If the information you have gathered indicates that behaviours that challenge or distress are shown by the person when they are in noisy environments, can these be removed from the person's usual routines? Can we offer noise-cancelling headphones to wear when in these situations? Can the person attend these places when they are quieter?
- Are there enough people who are skilled in person-centred approaches?
- Do people communicate with the person in their preferred way?
- Are there supports for maintaining and improving health and well-being and other quality-of-life domains? (See Chapter 1.)
- If the information says the person's preferred mode of communication is written instruction rather than verbal, can the person have easy access to an electronic tablet on which to type? Can they be given a pad and pen? Can others ensure they also use written instructions?
- If the analysis indicates that the person is likely to engage in behaviours that challenge when they are on their own as a means of accessing interaction, can we ensure they have a higher amount of interaction from others? Can we advocate for more support hours?

Developing new skills and opportunities

We should always begin with skills and opportunities the person would want to learn and that they would find *fun* to do.

Again, review the information that has been gathered. Pay particular attention to any skills assessments that indicate areas of interest. Consider the person's preferences. Are there any activities/tasks that increase independence but also involve items the person enjoys (i.e. doing the dishes, since the person likes water; recycling, since the person likes to sort items; play a musical instrument, as the person would like to learn)?

There also needs to be a consideration for any coping and tolerance plans that need to be implemented. These are skills that can help the person to manage difficult situations. It's important to remember that if the situations can simply be removed from the person's life this should be done (i.e. if they don't like busy shops, enable them to shop online or at smaller stores). If, however, there are situations that cause distress which cannot be removed or are linked to the person's preferences (they fear dogs, for example, but enjoy going for country walks, or they do not like crowds but enjoy live football games), strategies may need to be implemented to support the person to manage these situations.

Within the developing news skills and opportunities element of the MEBS plan, it is also critical to consider the function of behaviour. Plans should then be developed that support the person to meet the function and message of the behaviour, meaning behaviours that challenge are less likely to occur.

Examples:

- If the assessment shows that the person wants access to others' attention but has no means other than self-injurious behaviour to gain it, can we teach the person to sign, write or gesture (patting chair) to indicate they would like others to come and speak with them? Can we then teach staff to respond to these methods of communication immediately and consistently? Can we ensure the person has people who engage with the person routinely?
- If the assessment shows that the person engages in behaviours that challenge to get others to leave them alone, can they be taught to sign, write or gesture to get others to leave? Can those around them be taught to understand this and remove themselves?
- If the assessment shows that the person engages in behaviours that challenge to get access to snacks or drinks, can the person be taught to make their own snacks and drinks when they would like them?

 Enabling Capable Environments © Pavilion Publishing and Media Ltd and its licensors 2024.

Prevention/focused support strategies

Focused support strategies also need to be considered when developing the MEBS plan. As these plans can be linked to the function of behaviour, this must be considered as well as the motivating operations/setting events and the person's likes and dislikes.

Examples:

- Things the person does not like or which can upset them should be permanently or temporarily removed, if they are known (i.e. specific words, phrases, tasks).
- Time spent doing activities the person enjoys or with people they enjoy being with can be increased.
- If we know the function of behaviour, we can make sure they have less reason to rely on it until they have a better means of communicating.
- Remember, some of these strategies may be temporary until new environmental strategies and/or new skills are developed.

Resolution strategies

As discussed earlier, resolution strategies are designed to respond to incidents safely and rapidly when they occur. If we want to de-escalate a situation as quickly as possible, providing the need the person is seeking will do this. It is important to know the function of behaviour as well as the situations in which these occur, to have available, and then provide this as a resolution response. For more information, please see Chapter 11.

MEBS example

Here we will highlight key findings from a functional assessment for Jane and will provide an example of how a MEBS plan could be developed to meet her needs. Please note, an assessment will provide much more detailed information (see Chapter 10); we have used key points as an illustrative example.

Jane is 22 and lives in a shared flat with someone she went to school with. She moved here six months ago. Her family live nearby and visits at weekends; the team don't encourage weekday visits as they believe Jane needs to be more independent of her family.

Enabling Capable Environments © Pavilion Publishing and Media Ltd and its licensors 2024.

The assessment has shown:

- Noisy spaces have always been difficult for Jane.
- When Jane was young, she would always hide in cupboards at parties.
- Jane will regularly place her hands over her ears.
- Jane likes to listen to loud music, but only on her own and only when she asks for it to be put on. Jane can become distressed if staff do not switch the songs or put the music off when she has asked.
- Jane used to use Makaton at school. Her staff team do not understand Makaton but do think Jane tries to use some signs.
- Jane likes things done in a particular way and can become distressed when routines are changed.
- Jane is discouraged from doing household tasks. Others feel she needs these tasks to be done for her as she becomes distressed when things are not done in a set way and the kitchen can be dangerous.
- When engaging in tasks, Jane does not like verbal instructions.
- All of Jane's staff do the household activities in different orders and at different times of the day.

The hypothesised function of Jane's behaviour is summarised as 'Escape': to get others to leave her alone, get away from distressing situations, or when routines do not go as planned.

- The message of her behaviour is:
  - I don't know what's going to happen.
  - I feel overwhelmed.
  - I need to do things in the right order.

Using the information from the assessment and the quality-of-life domains, the participants developed a MEBS plan – Table 10.7 (please note, this is a synopsis of a MEBS plan and each element will need a detailed written plan to support it; developing support plans is detailed in Chapter 8).

 Enabling Capable Environments © Pavilion Publishing and Media Ltd and its licensors 2024.

Table 10.7: MEBS plan

Proactive strategies			Resolution strategies
Environmental strategies	**Skills teaching & opportunities**	**Prevention strategies**	**Function-based non-aversive reactive strategies**
Physical environment: ■ Storage areas to have a picture on the front so everyone knows where items should be. ■ Noise-cancelling headphones to be always available. ■ Garden area to have new seating area & plants. Interpersonal environment: ■ All staff to be trained in Makaton. ■ Family contact whenever Jane chooses. Service environment: ■ Written and visual steps of how Jane likes tasks to be done.	■ Plan an open-air concert. General skills: ■ Learn to make dinner for her friends and family. Functionally Equivalent skills: ■ Learning signs for 'stop' and 'help me'. Functionally Related skills: ■ Using a planner to show staff what she would like to do and when.	Antecedents: ■ Follow strategies in the sensory profile assessment. ■ Model going for a walk to the garden when Jane shows signs things are too much. Increase of preferred events: ■ Sign up to one-month free downloads from a music provider. Jane can then access it whenever she needs to. ■ Daily call to a family member to keep connected and not feel isolated.	■ Ask Jane to show you how she would like a task completed. ■ Direct to something she prefers to do. ■ Begin to sign or sing her favourite song. ■ Using Makaton to sign 'see you later' and leave the room. ■ Use of voice-activation setting on music to turn it off.

Philosophy and values:	Coping skills:	Reinforcement schedule:	
■ Team uses principles of PCAS to enhance opportunities to engage in activities i.e. the person having choice & control. ■ Person-centred plan is developed into person-centred actions. ■ The values of the team are aspirational to people having a good quality of life and committed to removing barriers to achieving this.	■ Using the sensory garden as a quiet space when the environment is too busy or noisy. ■ Using headphones in busy areas i.e. buses, shops.	■ Developed to increase the use of signing for assistance.	

 Enabling Capable Environments © Pavilion Publishing and Media Ltd and its licensors 2024.

Thinking space

Think about developing a MEBS plan, who might be able to help you create one?

- The person themselves.
- Friends of the person.
- Family of the person.
- Support staff.
- Teachers.

People who know the person will be useful collaborators in creating a MEBS plan. Remember to use the information and analysis you have completed.

Think about how you might gain their feedback and views:

- Could you arrange a meeting with everyone?
- Could you send requests for ideas and draw these together?
- Could you send suggestions and ask for votes and feedback?

Implementing the MEBS plan

It is not enough to simply create an overview of a MEBS plan. Each strategy within the plan will require instructions and guidance for others to follow on a day-to-day basis. Strategies that require simple changes, such as soundproofing or alterations to lighting, should be completed and then added to the person's support plan/Individual Education Plan, detailing that these requirements should be met in all areas of the person's life. All other plans should be developed into written instructions, showing others how to implement them in practice (see Chapter 8 for more information on creating new skills plans and templates).

When introducing any new plans into the person's support, it may be important to consider how many new plans are introduced at any given time. Too many new strategies being implemented could be overwhelming for both the person and the people who support them. It may be beneficial to stagger the introduction of plans, with the plans that are likely to have the most impact on the person's quality of life being introduced earlier. Plans such as reactive and focused supports may have an immediate effect on the person's and other's safety and should likely be introduced during the first stage.

Enabling Capable Environments © Pavilion Publishing and Media Ltd and its licensors 2024.

In addition to providing written instructions for each new plan, training, coaching and mentoring should be offered. This will ensure everyone is confident in implementing the plan and that they are doing so correctly (procedural fidelity). In Chapter 5, we discuss that the role of a practice leader is to help people move from being able to say what needs to be done (verbal competence), where they can describe what they should do and why, to doing it in practice (practice competence), where people do what is needed (LaVigna *et al*, 1994).

This is a form of scaffolding, to move from knowing what to do to doing what needs to be done. Typically, teams need support to move from reading a support plan. They need the practice lead to spend time with them, clarifying, coaching and providing feedback at each of the steps illustrated below.

Figure 10.2: Scaffolding support plan competency (Five tiers to competency)

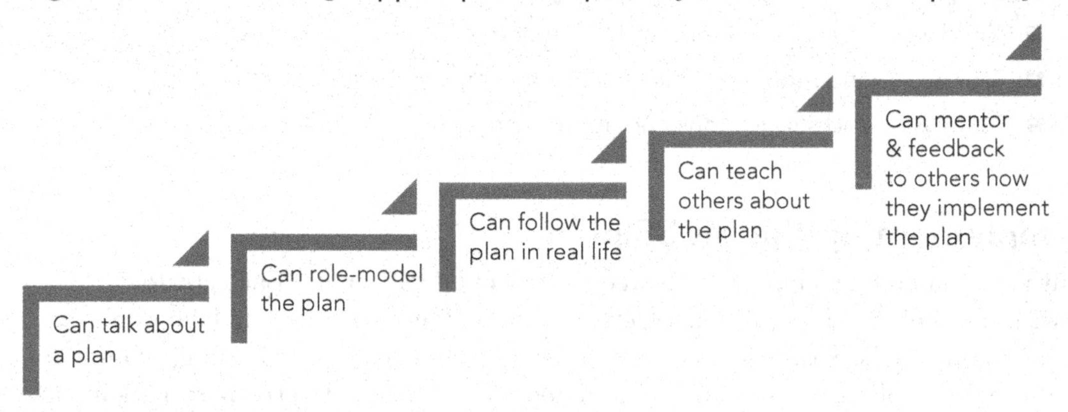

(Adapted from LaVigna *et al*, 1994. For more information, Chapter 5.)

These stages involve:

1. **Instruction:** The person/people who developed the plan should provide clear written instructions on what to do, and the team can articulate the key points of the plan and why they are needed.
2. **Modelling:** The person/people who developed the plan should show others how to do it. This could be through role-play or through completing the skills in practice. Those who will be implementing the plan should be able to role-play it.
3. **Practice:** People can do the plan in practice with coaching and feedback. The person who developed the plan should observe the person learning the skill and provide feedback on their performance. Feedback should be focused on both areas that require more work, as well as areas that have been achieved well.

 Enabling Capable Environments © Pavilion Publishing and Media Ltd and its licensors 2024.

4. **Teaching:** Team members who are now skilled in the plan can teach others the plan (step one).
5. **Mentoring:** Team members who are skilled in the plan can provide support and feedback to others to implement the plan (using the above four steps).

Thinking space

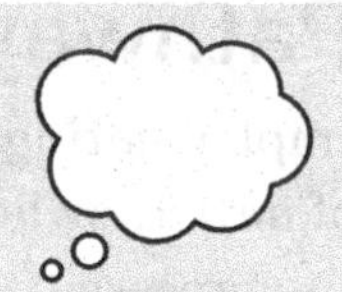

Think about a time you were learning a new skill. What helped you to understand and implement that skill well?

- Were written instructions helpful?
- Would images help you to understand the steps involved?
- Would seeing someone else doing the skill help you to learn? Could this be in practice or through video?
- Was it helpful to practice in a classroom before trying it in practice?

Think about what type of feedback helped you to enhance your skills and make changes where needed:

- How was this feedback communicated to you?
- Would written feedback have helped?
- Who would you like to provide that feedback?
- Would someone showing you again help?

Supporting a monitoring MEBS

After implementing MEBS plans, there is also a need to monitor its implementation. A periodic service review (PSR) is an effective method for doing this. PSR standards need to be developed for each MEBS plan. For more information on developing a PSR, please see Chapter 7.

Enabling Capable Environments © Pavilion Publishing and Media Ltd and its licensors 2024.

Pathways to success

Implementing and maintaining a MEBS plan will take time, effort, and likely a lot of new knowledge and skills. Here are some ways to support yourself throughout the process:

- You may be conducting a functional assessment and implementing a MEBS plan for the first time. Ensure you give yourself enough time to learn the new information and skills before conducting these.
- If doing this for the first time, we recommend gaining support from someone who has skills and experience in supporting others to implement a MEBS plan.
- Conducting a functional assessment and implementing a MEBS plan will not happen overnight. Give yourself enough time to do this well.
- Organisation will be key. Plan each step of the process and schedule when you will complete each part in advance.
- Plan your diary and the tasks with someone else who can help you consider additional pressures or factors that may affect each task.
- Keep things on track, we have said this can take time but you also need a plan that works for you. Ensure you have a mentor to help you keep on track and prioritise actions.
- Always think about the elements of the process in collaboration with others, this helps to have a more meaningful plan and enhances the quality of the recommendations.

Discussion questions

Below are some possible questions you are likely to be asked or you will ask during the process of developing and implementing MEBS plans.

1. **Won't this process take too long? We need plans now.** If there are immediate safety risks, temporary plans can be introduced as prevention strategies and access to the things the person likes can be increased, but remember, if we want to make long-term changes that meet the person's needs and increase their quality of life, the MEBS process is essential. Research has

 Enabling Capable Environments © Pavilion Publishing and Media Ltd and its licensors 2024.

shown that multi-elemental approaches, based on functional assessment, are key to meaningful change.

2. **What if there isn't enough time to train staff in the plans? Can they not just read through them?** MEBS plans may not be complex but they may include novel skills and approaches that the team are not familiar with. Attempting to transfer knowledge from written work into practice can be difficult. We need to take into consideration everyone's learning styles and think about the training and support people need, refer to the scaffolding of support plans competency discussion earlier in this chapter and Chapter 5. It is likely that, without training, others will not implement new plans in practice.
3. **I think I know what the function is, is a functional assessment really needed?** A functional assessment must be completed. If you were to incorrectly identify the function of behaviour (which is very easy to do), the plans that are developed could be ineffective (and therefore a waste of time and resources) or could make things worse. For example, imagine you wrongly assumed the person was trying to communicate that they wanted your time and attention, so you implement plans that ensure they have lots of it, and when they are distressed you provide additional time and attention. However, if the person was in fact communicating that they wanted to be left alone or have time to themself, your interventions could escalate the situation and further distress the person.

Far-reaching benefits of MEBS

Many of the difficulties people with an intellectual disability face are due to the barriers and attitudes they face. When approached from a human rights perspective, the MEBS model helps to decrease these barriers by enhancing participation skills and addressing interpersonal and physical environmental deficiencies (Doody, 2009). It is designed to enhance decision-making and choice (increasing empowerment) and increase skills that allow the ability to exercise rights to fairness and equality. As the MEBS model works towards achieving the above-stated rights, this ensures accountability, another key human rights standard (Doody, 2009).

Conclusion

Multi-element behaviour support (MEBS) is a structured model that supports the delivery of PBS (Doody, 2009). MEBS incorporates a range of proactive and reactive strategies which, together, increase quality of life, decrease the likelihood of future behaviours that challenge, and support the safe management of behavioural episodes (McClean & Grey, 2012b).

LaVigna & Willis (2005) stress that the focus of research and application in PBS may have relied on individual interventions, leading to a misunderstanding of PBS as a set of standalone interventions that disregard the broader context and outcomes. They propose that the integrated MEBS model, involving a focus being placed on several interventions which address different areas of a person's life, is required to fully understand and support change.

Behaviour support plans are only regarded as valid if they achieve the outcome of increasing quality of life (increasing choice, control, opportunities, meaningful relationships and community access), enhancing skills, and reducing behaviours that challenge (O'Brien & O'Brien, 1991).

LaVigna & Willis (2005) developed the multi-element behaviour support plan. This plan is based on a functional assessment and contains both proactive and reactive strategies that meet the function of behaviour, which helps to address quality-of-life deficiencies and decreases behaviours that challenge.

Proactive strategies are designed to make changes to behaviour over a long time. These are the strategies that have a real impact on quality of life and future engagement in behaviour. There are three categories of proactive strategies within the MEBS model:

- Environmental strategies.
- New skills and opportunities strategies.
- Prevention strategies.

Resolution strategies are designed to manage incidents safely and quickly when they occur. No learning or teaching is designed to take place within the reactive strategies. This is specifically reserved for proactive strategies.

Research has shown that frontline staff and managers can develop and implement MEBS in practice. This research has shown significant improvements to the quality of life for the individual and improvements to the quality of support and lives of people supporting the person. In addition to such improvements, there is a decrease in the frequency, duration and severity of behaviours that challenge.

 Enabling Capable Environments © Pavilion Publishing and Media Ltd and its licensors 2024.

Chapter 11: The Role of Resolution Strategies

'We need to stop hurting people in the name of helping them.'
Herb Lovett (1996)

Chapter contents:

- Understanding and responding to behaviours that challenge.
- What is meant by reactive strategies?
- Understanding the alignment fallacy and barriers to resolution.
- The role of episodic severity.
- First resort strategies – what are they and why they are important?
- Non-aversive reactive strategies – what they are and why they are important.

Learning outcomes

After reading this chapter and completing the suggested activities and reflection, the reader should be able to:

- Understand the role of reactive strategies and resolution strategies.
- Recognise the need for planned responses in supporting people during a time of crisis.
- Identify person-centred responses to resolving episodes of behaviours that challenge.
- Recognise the need for attuned responses in the support of people with an intellectual disability.
- Develop non-aversive reactive support strategies.

Introduction

In Chapter 9, we outlined what we mean by challenging behaviour. Most UK policy and guidance documents use the term 'challenging behaviour', but we acknowledge that there are variations to this term. In Chapter 7 we outlined the historical contexts around the terminology of challenging behaviour and the importance of understanding why behaviour occurs or does not occur to use this understanding to better support people.

This chapter continues with a similar theme: when we understand the messages of behaviour, we are better placed to support people in a way that is helpful to them. Some support systems need to recognise that this understanding of behaviour and how it informs what we do applies not only to the proactive strategies of support (see Chapter 7) but equally, if not more importantly, to the reactive strategies we employ.

The Herb Lovett quote at the beginning of this chapter is from a book entitled *Learning to Listen* (1996). The chapter summarises a concern from Lovett that processes and policies of that time were beginning to legitimise the use of harmful and aversive practices for people with an intellectual disability, i.e., 'hurting people'. Examples of the practices referred to were physical restraint, methods of coercion and control over the individual, and that such practices were being 'justified' in the context of risk management, i.e., 'helping' the person. Such concerns remain valid today.

In our clinical work, we often ask people:

- Is your response to someone's behaviour aimed at helping the person or trying to control them?
- When someone is at their most distressed or at the most risk of hurting themselves or others, would a response *attuned to the person's needs* be more likely to be effective?

A logical response would be 'Yes' to the first question, of course, we would try to be helpful. However, we often find that the answer to our second question is met with more muted responses. People have become so focused on managing risk, perceived or otherwise, that what the person needs can be overlooked or even ignored in pursuing a risk assessment.

 Enabling Capable Environments © Pavilion Publishing and Media Ltd and its licensors 2024.

What is meant by 'reactive strategy'?

> *'The role of a reactive strategy is to keep people safe in the here and now; not with an intent to influence change in the future.'* (LaVigna & Willis, 2005)

The first part of this statement will be a familiar concept to many as it is a critical component of policy, guidance and training in supporting people with an intellectual disability where there is a need to keep people safe when behaviours that challenge occur. Furthermore, from a practical perspective, we should keep people safe if someone is hurting themselves or others.

However, this concern with what we do now and how it may impact the future occurrence of behaviour is fraught with misconceptions. Examples include a misunderstanding that what you do in response to challenging behaviour may reinforce such behaviour or a belief that certain types of behaviour need to be responded to in a certain way. Another example we hear about in our clinical practice is that people with an intellectual disability must learn not to behave in a certain way and consequences must follow these behaviours to ensure this.

All these dilemmas are essential discussions, and we will address each of these misconceptions in turn as we progress through this chapter. In this section, we will firmly ground ourselves in what we mean by keeping people safe here and now.

Case study

Consider this as an illustrative example:

You share an office with a colleague; let us call her Shelly. You know that Shelly has recently been promoted from support worker to senior support worker. She loves her new role but is struggling with some of the new administration responsibilities that come with the job. Her line manager calls her, asks why she is late sending out next month's staff rota and asks that it be completed before the end of the day. Shelly hangs up the phone, throws all the paperwork from her desk into the air and places her head on her desk, saying, 'I just can't do this'.

- How would you respond in this scenario?
- What would you say? What would you do?

Now let us consider Jake:

Jake lives in a supported living service for people with an intellectual disability. Jake has not had much sleep, and there is a new support worker he has never met in the kitchen. Jake sits at the table and the new support worker asks, 'Did you wash your hands before sitting down?' Jake lifts the cereal box, empties it all over the table, makes a loud noise and puts his head on it.

- How would Jake be responded to in this scenario?
- What would you say? What would you do?

Thinking space

In both scenarios, Shelly and Jake appear to have had someone make a request that overwhelmed them. Even without an assessment (functional or otherwise), we can consider our response.

Shelly's colleagues would likely respond with some or all the following:

- Ask if she is okay.
- Offer to help.
- Offer a reassuring pat on the shoulder.
- Make her some tea.
- Offer to do the rota for her.
- The list goes on.

What is critical here is that, as a colleague, you see something is not working and that the person needs something, and you offer to help.

Now consider what the list for Jake would look like as someone with an intellectual disability supported in a shared living environment. Would the same list that was created for Shelly come up, or would it look different?

- Jake is told to clean up the mess.
- Jake is told to leave the kitchen.
- Jake is told he cannot go out as his behaviour is too challenging.
- Staff press an alarm so other support staff move Jake away from the cereal.
- The list could go on.

Why would such different approaches be pursued?

 Enabling Capable Environments © Pavilion Publishing and Media Ltd and its licensors 2024.

In Jakes's scenario, the team may be more concerned with the future effects of their response. For example, Jake must learn that he cannot make a mess. Alternatively, Jake's new support worker could be concerned that Jake has previously hit people. Here, the focus is on what has happened previously as an indicator of what might happen in the future. This concern with what has happened or what may happen in the future is not the focus of a reactive strategy.

Remember, a reactive strategy aims to keep people safe in the here and now, and this is typically best done by responding to what the person needs.

Think about what responses you use when presented with behaviours that challenge:

- Are your responses based on keeping safe?
- Are your responses focused on what you think the person may need?
- Are you considering what the message of the behaviour is and using this to do something helpful in that specific situation?

If the answer is no, then consider why you are responding in the way you do and keep a note as you progress through this chapter.

Why do we get stuck working out how to respond?

Understanding the alignment fallacy

To the best of our knowledge, this term was first used in the context of reactive strategies by LaVigna & Willis in 2005. In this paper, the authors state that there is a misconception that the more severe someone's behaviour is, the more restrictive the practices need to be to manage it. They describe how our perceptions of what we face and our assumptions of risk can drive our responses (LaVigna & Willis, 2005).

A basic example of this is the myth that if someone is behaving in a certain way it must require a certain type of response. Some examples we have seen/heard about in our work include:

- Oh, he is big and strong we need to do…
- If I give in it will just teach them…
- They need to learn that they can't do…

Some of these arguments may seem well founded, for example perhaps a member of the team has been injured in the past or the person injured themself. All these scenarios can seem quite rational in the moment but are flawed when viewed through a lens of power and control over the person rather than through a lens of resolution/helping.

Exploring traditional approaches

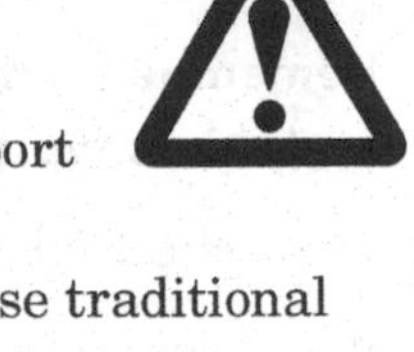

What we can see is often a tension between positive behaviour support reactive strategies and traditional approaches to responding to behaviour that is viewed as 'difficult', 'challenging' or 'naughty'. These traditional approaches can be more familiar to people. Consider your own experiences or upbringing – when you were late for school or didn't do your homework you may have received detention, when you took chips from your brother's plate without asking you didn't get ice cream for dessert… the list continues.

Such examples are often associated with myths about reinforcement, for example, that people should not get something they like after they have done something incorrect because this will reinforce the behaviour. However, we should remind ourselves what the purpose of a reactive strategy is. It is to bring about a resolution as quickly and as safely as possible, therefore we should not be concerning ourselves with issues about reinforcement for two reasons. Firstly, the use of reinforcement (the introduction or removal of something to *increase* a behaviour) happens in our proactive strategies (more detail in Chapter 8 and Chapter 10). Secondly, people can be confused about where and when to teach skills. For example, people think the crisis situation is the time to teach about behaviour, but it is not. This may be when the person is most distressed. Think about a time when you were distressed, would this have been the best time to teach you a new skill to better meet your needs? Finally, the issue of whether to reinforce behaviour or not should be irrelevant in a crisis as our proactive plans should already address people having access to what they need and want, irrespective of their behaviour, so these things will not be reinforcing in a crisis.

We will walk you through some scenarios that illustrate these points. Our intention is not to sensationalise people's behaviour or, indeed, to diminish the seriousness of some behaviour, we are merely making some key points to consider about supporting people in a person-centred way.

 Enabling Capable Environments © Pavilion Publishing and Media Ltd and its licensors 2024.

As an example, let's return to Jake and the empty box of cereal. What we know from this very brief scenario:

- Jake is tired.
- There is someone in his kitchen he doesn't know.
- He knows it's breakfast time as he can see the cereal box on the table.
- A question is posed to him which, by the tone, is presented more as an accusation.

Without doing a detailed assessment, it is possible to come up with strategies that can ensure the situation does not escalate and will likely defuse the situation calmly and safely.

- **Distraction**: Can you get the orange juice from the fridge? (This is his favourite drink.)
- **Communication**: Using active listening helps to solve problems – 'You look tired this morning; would you like to watch some TV and we can have breakfast in a while?'
- **Inject humour**: 'That's a lot of cereal – we might need two spoons!' Be careful not to appear sarcastic or appear to be making fun of the person.
- **Offer assistance**: 'Do you need some help to put this in a bowl?'
- **Give instruction**: 'Shall we make some toast?'

Roadblocks to resolution

Below, we have based these 'roadblocks' on a school setting, but the points are equally applicable to any setting. The responses outlined may seem typical, natural, traditional, and obvious responses to behaviour that presents as challenging, but from the perspective of resolving the situation, they can be roadblocks and could potentially make the situation worse (escalation). This risks the use of aversive and negative responses leading to stress and trauma for the individual and the team/family member trying to navigate the situation.

Some typical responses that get in the way of resolving situations are:

- **Ordering or telling the person what you think they should do**. Example: 'Stop complaining and get back to learning the spellings!'
- **Warning or use of threats**. Example: 'You'd better get your story writing finished if you expect to get to break time.'
- **Moralising, preaching, using 'should' statements**. Example: 'You should leave your personal problems out of the classroom.'
- **Advising, offering solutions or suggestions**. Example: 'I think you need to get a daily planner so you can organise your time better to get your homework finished.'
- **Teaching, lecturing and giving logical arguments**. Example: 'You better remember you only have until lunchtime to complete your project work.'

These next responses tend to communicate the person is at fault for the situation they are in/finding difficulty with:

- **Judging, criticising, disagreeing, blaming**. Example: 'You are lazy. You never do what you say you will.' Or, 'Seems like you got up on the wrong side of the bed today.'
- **Name-calling, stereotyping, labelling**. Example: 'Act your age. You are not at playschool,'
- **Interpreting, analysing, diagnosing**. Example: 'You don't understand what you need to do because you were talking too much to your friends when it was being explained.'

Other messages that seem like they are trying to make the person feel better but are denying there is a problem are:

- **Praising, agreeing and giving positive evaluations**. Example: 'You are a smart child. You can figure out a way to finish this project.'
- **Reassuring, sympathising, consoling, supporting**. Example: 'I know exactly how you are feeling. If you just begin, it won't seem so bad.'

To clarify, we are saying the above strategies are not recommended and may escalate a situation, making it worse. We are trying to illustrate the point that if we want to help resolve a situation, we need to know where the issue lies and offer practical support to overcome this, here and now.

 Enabling Capable Environments © Pavilion Publishing and Media Ltd and its licensors 2024.

Thinking space

- What if we knew why the person was behaving in the way that they were?
- What if we knew that how we respond may make things worse for a while?
- What if we knew that if we responded in a way that was helpful this episode would end quickly?

This last bullet point refers to what are known as first resort strategies and very often training programmes pay lip service to these approaches or assume that you already know how to do them.

Consider the plans you have that tell you how to respond in a crisis situation, do they cover the three bullet points above?

- If the answer is no, then how do you know what your first resort strategies are?
- How do you know what to do that will work?
- How do you know that what you do will not make things worse?

Attunement and regulation

What do we mean by being attuned to someone? Attunement is a nonverbal process of being with another person in a way that attends fully and responsively to that person (Schore & Schore, 2008).

When we are attuned to someone, we are trying to make sense of their emotions and needs. It's about making the person feel heard and understood and using this understanding to be helpful in that moment. In very simple terms, it's about 'tuning' into the person's experience.

It is also important that we are attuned with ourselves. We discussed this in more detail in Chapter 4 but here, in the context of resolution strategies, we need to be aware of our own emotions if we are going to be in a place of helping others. It is about our reactiveness to a person in that moment.

Thinking space

Reflect on the last time you were annoyed about something or were anxious about doing something new.

You come home to tell your partner all about it and they sit at the table scrolling through their phone.

- How do you feel?
- Would you say anything?
- What would your tone be?

Some of us might tell them to stop what they are doing and listen to us.

Some of us might become upset and cry.

Some of us might grab the phone and shout at them.

None of us would feel listened to or that what we had to say was important. In our relationships with others, we need to feel safe and feel listened to (especially) when we are upset or things are not working for us.

Some guiding principles on attunement:

- Being attuned means that your eyes, facial expressions, tone of voice, body language, etc. are sending signals back to the person that are sensed and felt as being supportive to them.
- Tune in to pick up all signals, clues and cues which can indicate how the other person is feeling. Use this information to best understand their emotional, psychological and physical state.
- Through attunement, we show that we are 'listening', 'seeing' and understanding the other person. Attuned responsiveness sends the message that 'I am here with you, I care about you, and I want to understand you'.

Regulation and co-regulation

Co-regulation involves creating a sense of safety so you can both work out what all these emotions mean and make sense of them. As this needs to be seen from the individual's perspective, this can take a bit of time to work through, but this time taken to understand what is going on and what the person needs from you is critical – it is reflective of the quote from Hughes *et al.* (2019) 'Connection before correction'.

 Enabling Capable Environments © Pavilion Publishing and Media Ltd and its licensors 2024.

Several services adapt the 'Zones of Regulation' (Kuypers, 2011) or 'the window of tolerance' (Siegel, 2012) as templates for helping to map someone's behaviour to a particular zone. These approaches can be quite helpful, but we would suggest some caution in how these are applied (this is discussed below). Both approaches helpfully outline how people's emotional states are reflected in 'zones' (Kuypers, 2011) or 'windows' (Siegel, 2012) of regulation or arousal. The zones or areas that sit outside feeling regulated or optimum tolerance are commonly referred to as hyperarousal and hypoarousal.

Figure 11.1: Emotional regulation ranges

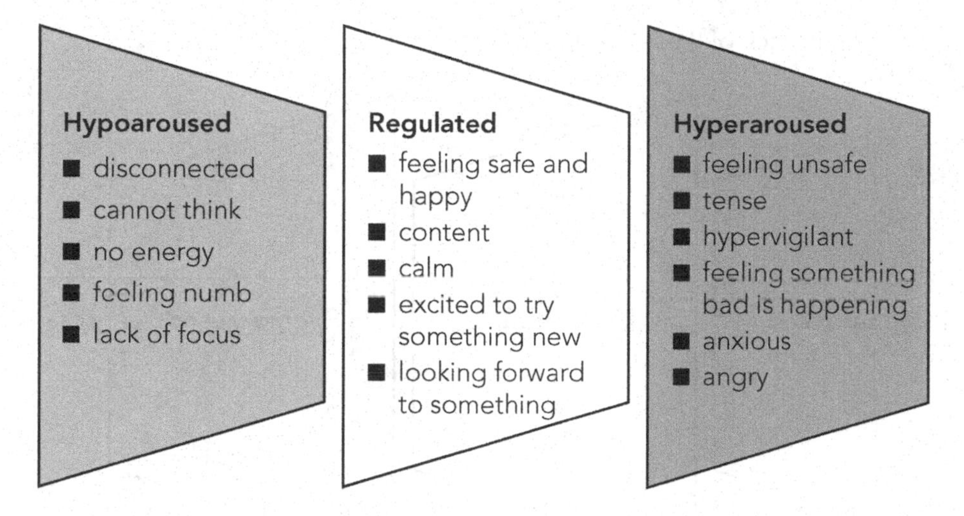

We would like to reiterate a point of caution about how these zones are interpreted and used in practice. For example:

- They should not be used as literal determiners of how someone is feeling – this is a suggested guide.
- People should not be referred to or talked about as being in the zones; in our practice, when visiting a service, we overheard someone being warned that an individual was having a 'red day' and we'd better be careful. This type of reference is dehumanising and does not help us to attune to what the person needs from us.
- There is no bad zone – as humans, we all experience moments of calm or feeling out of control.

Enabling Capable Environments © Pavilion Publishing and Media Ltd and its licensors 2024.

Thinking space

A short animation titled 'Panda's island of regulation' is available on Youtube. It is aimed at younger children, but the principal messages are about how we help people navigate through emotions proactively by teaching skills that help the person and reactively by helping to draw upon these skills during difficult times. The overarching theme is that we as the supporter have a key role in responding to people's needs in a humanistic and positive way.

Watch this video and then consider what you will do/say to co-regulate with someone you support in each of the emotional zones below.

What is your action in each of these areas?

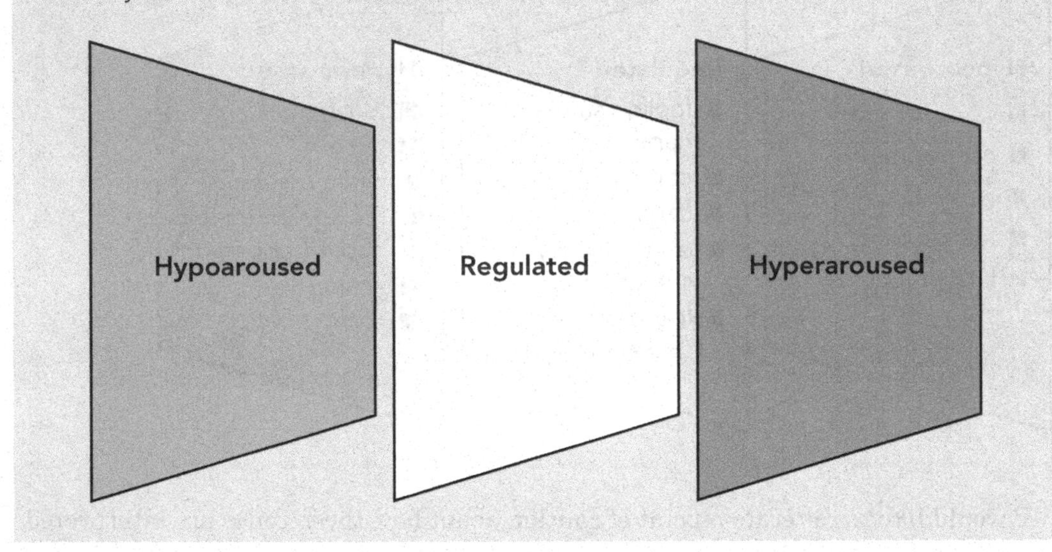

Humanistic approaches

In Chapter 1, we outlined what we mean by humanistic approaches and how these can shape our thinking and practices. For example, we discussed how we practice in a way that treats people as individuals and recognises that all people have the right to pursue personal development and aspirations; in other words, to be the best they can be and have the best life based on their preferences.

A humanistic approach also recognises that people's perceptions of the world differ and that their needs, wishes and aspirations are unique. If we start with the idea that people's perceptions and experiences of the world can be different to ours and

 Enabling Capable Environments © Pavilion Publishing and Media Ltd and its licensors 2024.

apply this to how we respond to behaviours that challenge, we may need to ask ourselves some key questions:

- How is the person experiencing the world just now?
- Are they frightened, angry, upset, overwhelmed or in pain?

The quote by Anne Donnellan *et al*. captures this moment-by-moment response and what actions we take to support someone:

> *'Our assumptions about a person's intention or meaning directly influence the way we respond moment to moment, the relationships we form and the support we give to people.'* (Donnellan, Hill & Leary, 2012)

By contrast, the following responses to behaviours that are presenting as challenging can typically include the following:

- Stop doing that.
- You need to learn you can't do that.
- Stop doing x or y will happen!

We refer to this as 'What is wrong with you thinking'. This is from a quote in Bloom (1995), who argues that there is a need to shift from responding to people's behaviour by asking 'what is wrong with you?', to asking 'what has happened to you?' This shift is designed to consider that all individuals have a history of experiences that can influence (whether intentionally or not) how people may respond in situations they find difficult or overwhelming.

Non-aversive reactive strategies (NARS)

Several chapters in this book have explored the importance of assessing and understanding why behaviour happens and why it may be challenging. We have directed you to think about what the messages behind such behaviour are. In this section, we were hoping you might continue this journey of understanding the messages of behaviour and how this understanding can inform your response at times when a person's behaviour has escalated to the point that they may cause harm to themselves or others, also referred to as a 'reactive strategy'. In addition, we will outline what you should do when the message/function of a behaviour is not understood.

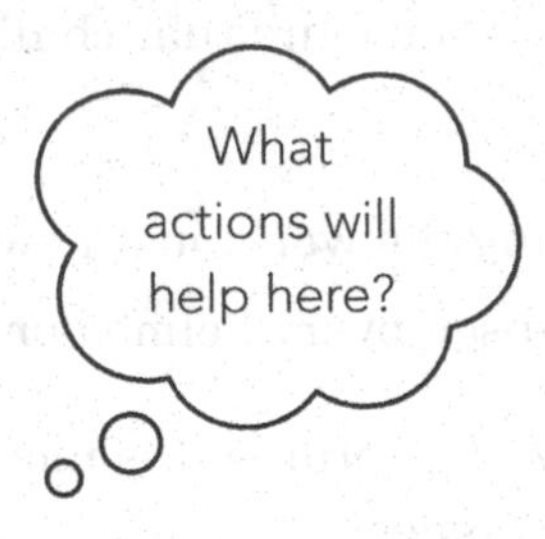

The term NARS was first outlined in the work of Crates and Spicer (2016) and Spicer and Crates (2016). In their work, they summarise NARS as being a way to respond to behaviour challenges or crises which does not involve the use of punishment or ways that the person would find aversive, for example, the use of restrictive practices. They outline two categories of NARS, the first being functionally based responses, where the function of behaviour has been assessed and summarised. The second is 'non-functionally based', where the reason for the behaviour is not understood.

What is being applied here is a way of viewing the person with dignity and respect. The purpose of reactive strategies is to bring about resolution as quickly and as safely as possible. We have already outlined how and why person-centred approaches are important in a reactive strategy, but the concept of safety does need to be explored in more detail. In our research (Hume *et al.*, 2021) we refer to the term 'episodic severity' which looks to measure the severity of each incident (LaVigna & Willis, 2005). This variable is the seriousness of the behaviour and its impact on the person and/or others. We must ask ourselves, is our response to behaviour going to escalate (increase the episodic severity) or resolve (decrease episodic severity)? Our goal is to always reduce the episodic severity (for more information on episodic severity, see Chapter 9).

Table 11.1 summarises key evidence-based strategies that can reduce episodic severity.

 Enabling Capable Environments © Pavilion Publishing and Media Ltd and its licensors 2024.

Table 11.1: NARS key strategies

Functionally based non-aversive reactive strategies (FB-NARS) ***Responding with an understanding of the function/message of behaviour***	Non-functionally based non-aversive reactive strategies (NARS) ***Responding without an understanding of the function/message of behaviour but in a person-centred/attuned way***
Message of behaviour: Seeking interaction/connection. ■ Active listening. ■ Provide individual. Attention/ Interaction. ■ Talk about their favourite subject. **Message of behaviour: Trying to meet a sensory need.** ■ Provide sensory activity. ■ Model accessing sensory experiences, for example, running in the garden, jumping on the trampoline, and blowing bubbles. **Message of behaviour: Trying to escape/ avoid something they find upsetting or unpleasant.** ■ Remove demands. ■ Encourage them to leave the area. ■ Move away from the person. ■ Practice calming techniques **Message of behaviour: Trying to get something tangible they want or need.** ■ Give the person what they want/ need. ■ Plan how they can get what they want/need if not immediately available. ■ Substitute with a close proximity, for example, they want to see their favourite person but they are not available, so call them, write a note for them, etc.	■ Active Listening. ■ Remove demands. ■ Distraction to a known and preferred activity/person. ■ Ask them to help you. ■ Facilitate problem-solving. ■ Facilitate coping strategies.

Enabling Capable Environments © Pavilion Publishing and Media Ltd and its licensors 2024.

Non-function-based reactive strategies

In our study (Hume *et al.*, 2021), the training component used the capable environment characteristics as a framework for developing reactive strategies. In this project, the team were able to identify general strategies (non-function-based) that were considered helpful in responding to a crisis situation for their focus person. These were strategies that were considered helpful in resolving a situation where an assessment of the function (message) of the behaviour had not been undertaken.

Some examples of these non-function-based reactive strategies (NARS) are provided below:

Table 11.2: NARS capable environments template plan

Characteristic	NARS Plan
Positive social interactions	Consider your tone of voice, your posture and the words you use. What messages do these give to the person? ■ Are you asking for ways to help the person? ■ Are you presenting with an open and friendly posture? ■ Do others smile at/with the person? ■ Do people talk to the person and ask them questions? ■ Do others have relaxed body language? ■ Does the person know you are there to support them? ■ Do you offer reassurance that everything is/will be okay? ■ Are you minimising noise and fuss so as not to embarrass the person, especially if there are other people around?

 Enabling Capable Environments © Pavilion Publishing and Media Ltd and its licensors 2024.

Support for communication	If the person is upset, think about how your communication style and what you are saying may need to change: ■ Do you need to use some prompts rather than speaking? ■ Do you need to stay quiet and just let the person vent for a bit? ■ Are you constructive in what you are saying, for example being positive 'Let's go and make some tea' rather than being negative 'Stop doing…'? ■ Can you introduce a topic the person likes to hear about or likes to join in with, for example, a favourite TV programme or an activity that is coming up such as a birthday?
Provision of opportunities for choice	In a crisis, is the person provided with choices? And are these are respected? ■ Are choices offered to the person using their preferred method of communication? ■ Are choices offered that maintain the person's dignity in a crisis? ■ Do others understand when some choices may overwhelm the person and how to limit this if appropriate?

Enabling Capable Environments © Pavilion Publishing and Media Ltd and its licensors 2024.

<table>
<tr>
<td>Personal care and health support</td>
<td>Are people aware of the signs and symptoms that suggest the person is unwell?
<ul>
<li>Do others (where appropriate) know the person's medical and health needs?</li>
<li>Are people clear about how to respond to these signs and symptoms, for example:
<ul>
<li>Access to pain relief?</li>
<li>Access to health professionals?</li>
<li>Access to other relief medication, for example hay fever, constipation, indigestion relief?</li>
</ul>
</li>
<li>If there are specific health needs, are others trained to support this (i.e., epilepsy, diabetes, etc.)?</li>
<li>Is the person able to communicate health or pain needs through their preferred method of communication? Can the person be directed to this during a crisis?</li>
<li>Is there easy access to communication aids that support the person's ability to communicate their health needs? If not, how can you make this more accessible? Particularly in crisis situations.</li>
</ul>
</td>
</tr>
</table>

Enabling Capable Environments © Pavilion Publishing and Media Ltd and its licensors 2024.

Function-based reactive strategies

Group activity

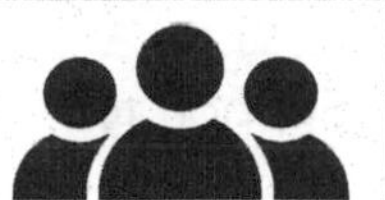

Using Table 11.3, below, consider each of the components in turn and tailor some function-based non-aversive strategies for an individual you support.

Remember, function-based non-aversive reactive strategies are aimed at addressing, where possible, the message (the function of behaviour).

You should ensure you have correctly assessed the function of behaviour (see Chapter 9).

Table 11.3: Capable environments – function-based NARS template

Characteristic	The message (function) of the behaviour is	Likely function-based NARS
Support for communication		
Characteristic	**The message (function) of the behaviour is**	**Likely function-based NARS**
Support for participation in meaningful activity		
Characteristic	**The message (function) of the behaviour is**	**Likely function-based NARS**
Provision of consistent and predictable environments which honour personalised routines and activities		

Enabling Capable Environments © Pavilion Publishing and Media Ltd and its licensors 2024.

Characteristic	The message (function) of the behaviour is	Likely function-based NARS
Support to establish and/ or maintain relationships with family and friends		
Characteristic	**The message (function) of the behaviour is**	**Likely function-based NARS**
Provision of opportunities for choice		
Characteristic	**The message (function) of the behaviour is**	**Likely function-based NARS**
Personal care and health support		
Characteristic	**The message (function) of the behaviour is**	**Likely function-based NARS**
Provision of an acceptable physical environment		

Conclusion

Ginott (1993) reflected that:

> 'I've come to the frightening conclusion that I am the decisive element in the classroom. It's my daily mood that makes the weather. As a teacher, I possess a tremendous power to make a child's life miserable or joyous. I can be a tool of torture or an instrument of inspiration. I can humiliate or humor, hurt or heal…it is my response that decides whether a crisis will be escalated or de-escalated, a child humanized or de-humanized.'

Enabling Capable Environments © Pavilion Publishing and Media Ltd and its licensors 2024.

The above quote is based on the author's experiences in a school setting, yet in our clinical experience, the key messages apply in multiple service settings and, indeed, in people's homes. In Chapter 1 we discussed how people with intellectual disability are often reliant on others to support them to navigate their way through barriers in their daily lives. Those who are relied upon are often custodians of people's rights, dignity, and autonomy; in many instances, people who provide support are custodians in the context of being protectors of these rights or advocates and champions. These are highly influential and, to an extent, powerful roles in a person's life, and caution is required. It is important in this role not to become a warden or judge of these rights based on some misconception that individuals with an intellectual disability are only entitled to these rights if they conform to a misguided perception of how they should behave in particular circumstances.

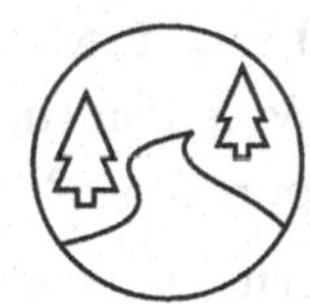

Paving the way to success

To summarise, we would advocate that all reactive strategies are based on the following principles:

- We respond to crisis situations with empathy and compassion.
- Our thoughts are focused on doing something that is intentionally helpful.
- Approaches are grounded in person-centred approaches.
- Quality assurance systems, for example, training and supervision, consider the support team's need to support approaches such as attunement and non-aversive reactive strategies.
- Evidenced-based approaches are used to support an understanding of behaviour.

Causton *et al.* (2015) summarise that:

'Each inclusive educator can reflect upon current practices and implement more humanistic supports. This is achieved by embracing strategies which value behavioural diversity within the classroom and support the whole student. Truly connecting and treating ALL students with dignity and respect will prove to be the most effective behavioural support for inclusive teachers allowing all students to focus on learning.'

Enabling Capable Environments © Pavilion Publishing and Media Ltd and its licensors 2024.

Final thoughts

This chapter has focused on non-aversive reactive strategies. We acknowledge that many services are trained in the use of restrictive practices and therefore we will provide some comment on their use. We would ask that all service providers who use restrictive practices consider the following points:

- All restrictive practices should be used as a last resort, be proportionate, and be used for the shortest time possible.
- Being proportionate and being for the shortest time possible means bringing about safety and resolution as quickly as possible. We have already demonstrated that the use of restrictive practices can escalate a situation and make things worse.
- If restrictive practices are the last resort, what are your first resort strategies, and how and when is training provided on these first resort strategies? How do you assess competence in these approaches?
- Managing risk – the episodic severity of each incident should be a key indicator of the effectiveness of reactive strategies; if it is increasing then the reactive strategies are likely to be aversive.
- All countries in the UK and most other countries have clear legislation about capacity and consent. These laws aim to ensure that the rights of people with an Intellectual Disability are upheld. For many people with an intellectual disability, there will be procedures in place to protect them from financial abuse and ensure they have access to health care, but we should also consider **assent**. This involves treating people with respect and compassion and ensuring that support does not cause harm. Withdrawing assent is an expression of unwillingness to participate and should be a right that is honoured.

When we say that services uphold human rights and have respect for the individual, these values are of even more importance during a crisis when a person is at their most distressed.

Enabling Capable Environments © Pavilion Publishing and Media Ltd and its licensors 2024.

Chapter 12: Evidence-based practice – what we should see

'The greatest challenge for any innovation lies at this point: in the move from the first exemplars to widespread implementation'.
(Mansell *et al.*,1994)

Chapter contents:

- Introduction.
- A guide for families.
- A guide for those directly supporting individuals with intellectual disabilities.
- A guide for organisational managers.
- A guide for commissioners and regulatory bodies.
- A guide to recommended training and consultation.
- Concluding note.

Introduction

The purpose of this book has been to present a unified framework for good practice that encourages a creative, flexible and effective structure of support delivery and training. The unified framework reflects a personalised system of support grounded in a humanistic approach and emphasises understanding and responding to support needs rather than focusing on challenging behaviour. In our unified framework, we advocate that quality of life is the foundation upon which person-centred supports are built, and is used as the primary criterion in evaluating this support. Applying a unified framework can improve service design and delivery for people with intellectual disabilities. However, more importantly, it improves an individual's quality of life by delivering more personalised support.

In Chapter 1, we presented a unified framework of support (Figure 12.1) that moves beyond an ecological perspective and considers a more holistic and humanistic understanding of people's life goals, and builds support systems accordingly. This concluding chapter will use this framework to guide what good support should look like for the many stakeholders involved in services, including those providing the support, those in charge of services, those who inspect and commission services, and the families of those receiving support. The authors of this book hope that it proves a valuable addition to the literature around quality-of-life improvement and a practical guide to understanding and implementing the many factors that lead to this improvement.

Figure 12.1: A unified approach to person-centred supports

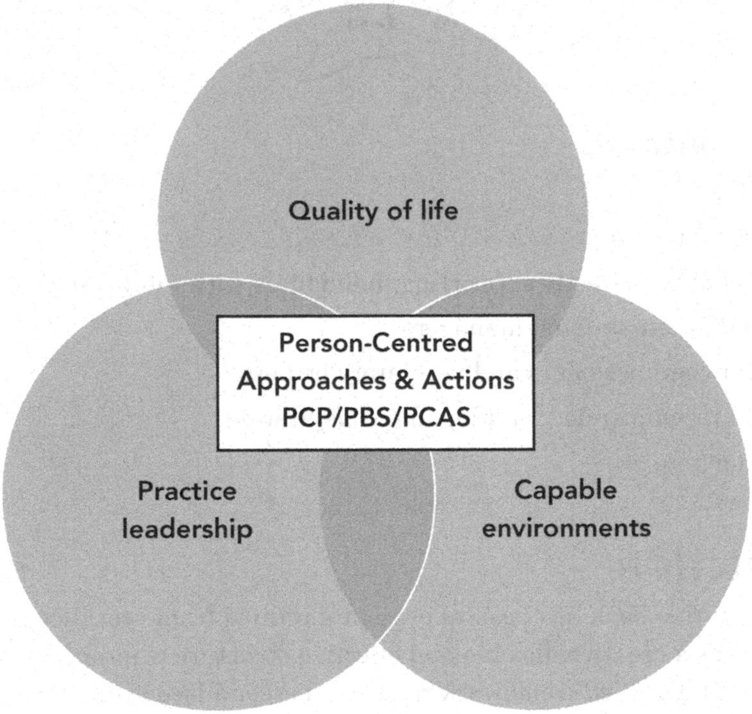

When there is a focus on quality of life, combined with effective practice leadership, based on a supportive framework such as capable environments, person-centred approaches and person-centred action can be facilitated.

 Enabling Capable Environments © Pavilion Publishing and Media Ltd and its licensors 2024.

A guide for families

Table 12.1 will provide families with a guide to the supports and systems that services should have in place to improve the quality of life of those receiving support and the support provided to family members.

Table 12.1: A guide for families

Quality of life	Practice leadership	Capable environments	Person-centred approaches and actions
Support for your family member is based on the principles of human rights, inclusion, equity and self-determination. Families are involved in the co-production of assessments and PBS plans, and other personalised plans, with the aim of improving their physical, emotional and psychological well-being, quality of life and enhancing personalised supports of family members.	The focus of practice leadership is on quality-of-life outcomes for your family member and that these are congruent with the principles of active support, which in turn influence how staff act in practice.	Staff supporting your family member use a capable environments plan which enhances support, for example: ■ Communication methods that meet the person's needs and preferences. ■ Increasing choice and control in all areas of the person's life. ■ Supporting engagement and participation at a pace and in a way that is right for the person. ■ Listening to the person and understanding their needs, wishes and goals.	Your family member has a person-centred plan (PCP) and the plan results in actions that are about their life and reflect what is possible and not what is available. The people supporting your family member routinely respond with empathy and compassion and in a crisis situation their thoughts are focused on 'doing something that is intentionally helpful'.

Enabling Capable Environments © Pavilion Publishing and Media Ltd and its licensors 2024.

		■ Ensuring that staff are skilled in providing the necessary personalised support your family member needs and that they are supported by the organisation to implement and evaluate this.	The people supporting your family member draw on the expert knowledge of the individual's family and friends to improve their understanding of what personalised support should look like and how it should be practiced. Where necessary, the team understand the general causes of behaviours that challenge and the specific influences on the individual's behaviour. They work with the family and others to develop plans to address these specific influences and ensure plans are focused on enhancing the person's quality of life.

A guide for support staff

Table 12.2 identifies the key systems and practices that support staff are responsible for delivering to provide personalised supports that are focused on improving the quality of life for individuals they work with.

Enabling Capable Environments © Pavilion Publishing and Media Ltd and its licensors 2024.

Table 12.2: A guide for support staff			
Quality of life	**Practice leadership**	**Capable environments**	**Person-centred approaches and actions**
Staff adopt a strengths-based approach to support, based on an individualised assessment of strengths and the desired living experience of the individual. Staff advocate for health equality and use necessary tools to do this, for example health action plans and healthcare passports. Staff teams adopt a proactive understanding of the impact health has on the person's life and overall well-being and quality of life.	Staff are involved in planning and implementing PCAS and work alongside practice leaders to improve the support they provide. Staff engage with coaching and mentoring support provided by practice leads. Staff are involved in the development and design of a system to evaluate practice i.e. periodic service review (PSR).	Staff provide daily support based on individualised plans using the capable environment appraisal. There is a specific focus on the eight characteristics which influence daily support. Staff teams use evaluation systems to ensure plans and practices are routinely evaluated, for example the use of a PSR associated with the person's individual plan(s)	Staff provide opportunities for engagement in meaningful activity and relationships. Staff work with individuals and their families to identify new opportunities, develop new skills and use the person's preferred method of learning to integrate them into their lives. Staff identify key areas of active support for an individual using the four principles of PCAS. Staff contribute to and follow advice and guidance contained within the person's personalised plans (support plans, PBS plans, skill teaching, etc.) Staff employ identified person-centred responses to resolving episodes of behaviours that challenge.

A guide for organisational managers

Table 12.3 provides organisational managers with a guide to identifying key models of support that focus on improved service delivery in the context of personalised supports and quality of life.

Table 12.3: A guide for organisational managers

Quality of life	Practice leadership	Capable environments	Person-centred approaches and actions
People in managerial roles are driven by the belief that individuals have the right to make choices and determine their goals and aspirations, irrespective of the level of intellectual disability. Support plans reflect the aspirations and needs of the individual and explicitly direct staff on how to provide support to meet these.	Organisational managers prioritise practice leadership, making it clear who within services holds this role, that the individual is aware of this, and has the skills and resources to perform the role effectively. Practice leaders support staff teams side-by-side through coaching, modelling and mentoring.	Managers ensure a capable environments appraisal has been completed to allow for the development of individual capable environment plans. Organisational managers prioritise an appraisal of the four elements of capable environments that can affect systems change (which ensure all other elements of a capable environment are implemented) namely: ■ Provision of an acceptable physical environment.	Quality assurance systems, for training and supervision consider the support teams need to support approaches such as humanistic personalised support, attunement and non-aversive reactive strategies. Managers facilitate regular supervision with staff. Supervision should be framed as supportive, educational and reflective.

 Enabling Capable Environments © Pavilion Publishing and Media Ltd and its licensors 2024.

Managers at every level, particularly senior managers, members of the board and trustees should prioritise the quality of life of the people they support and place a focus on this in everything they do. Quality of life should be a set agenda point at all meetings, targets should be set and clearly defined, and regular monitoring should be implemented to ensure this is achieved.	Barriers to providing good support are openly identified and discussed but the key is facilitating a process which identifies the enablers of good support. Managers are skilled at the type of support that they want to see.	■ Mindful skilled carers. ■ Effective organisational context. ■ Effective management and support.	Valuing and respecting staff's perspectives and making changes based on this is critical to enabling the team to embed such values in their day-to-day practices.

A guide for commissioners and regulatory bodies

Table 12.4 can serve as a guide to what evidence commissioners and regulatory bodies should request when measuring how effective services are at providing good quality supports.

Table 12.4: A guide for commissioners and regulatory bodies

Quality of life	Practice leadership	Capable environments	Person-centred approaches and actions
Services show evidence of: ■ Fostering the provision of individualised supports. ■ Furthering the development of evidence-based practices. ■ Encouraging the evaluation of personalised outcomes. ■ Providing a quality framework for continuous quality improvement.	Commissioners should request evidence which identifies who the practice leaders are in services, what support and training they have been provided, and the impact they are having (i.e. the impact they have on leading practices which improve people's quality of life and the processes which help this such as increased supervisions, observations, debriefings, etc.)	Commissioners and regulatory bodies identify that services are organised in a way that enables capable environments to ensure positive outcomes about participation, well-being and inclusion.	Commissioners and regulatory bodies identify that the individual being supported has a person-centred plan that reflects what is important to them, their preferences and what support is needed to reflect these. Commissioners and regulatory bodies identify that evidenced-based approaches are used to meet a person's behaviour support needs.

 Enabling Capable Environments © Pavilion Publishing and Media Ltd and its licensors 2024.

	Evidence should be available that measures quality of staff support and engagement, and improvements to the overall quality of services.		Commissioners and regulatory bodies identify evidence that personalised plans, including positive behaviour support plans, achieve the outcome of increasing quality of life (increasing choice, control, opportunities, meaningful relationships and community access), enhancing skills and reducing behaviours that challenge

A guide to recommended training and consultation

Table 12.5 aims to provide a guide to the core training needs which should be considered. It also identifies the need for collaboration and consultancy with external professionals to provide a holistic approach to personalised support needs.

Table 12.5: Recommended training and consultation

Quality of life	Practice leadership	Capable environments	Person-centred approaches and actions
Support teams use the 'Learning Disability and Human Rights: Practitioners Guide' as part of training, reflective supervision, team meetings, etc. as a way of ensuring the rights of people with a learning disability remain at the forefront of their practice. Staff should be provided with training on trauma-informed practices to better understand how our responses can be aversive or traumatising to the individuals we are supporting.	Managers ensure whole-environment training is available when implementing practice leadership. Specifically, the commitment to coaching, mentoring and supervising staff in the type of support they want to see being provided.	Core training should reflect the 12 components of a capable environment and that such training is personalised and relevant to the teams supporting the individual.	Specialist input should be used as needed to complement and enhance personalised support. This may be from health and social care teams who provide support from a range of professionals such as PBS specialists, psychiatrists, nurses, dieticians, speech and language therapists, etc.

Enabling Capable Environments © Pavilion Publishing and Media Ltd and its licensors 2024.

			A commitment to prioritising training that reflects the training needs of everyone involved in providing support. Examples of this include whole-environment training where the training provided is specific to the person's role. This acknowledges that everyone in the organisation has a focus on quality of life no matter what their role is.

Concluding note

Throughout this book, we have provided the reader with practical and realistic strategies for improving the quality of life of someone who requires the support of others. Advocating the need for person-centred approaches and an improved quality of life is not unique to this book; its uniqueness is situated in its ability to draw together the core components of creating and maintaining a high quality of services and quality of life under one unified framework that ensures a robust and systematic approach which is focused on delivering personalised support.

We have used our unified framework as a basis for good evidence-based support which encourages a creative, flexible and effective structure of support delivery and training. The unified framework reflects a personalised system of support that is grounded in a humanistic approach and aims to reflect a way of understanding and responding to support needs rather than focusing on what people perceive as being 'problem behaviour'. In our unified framework, we have advocated that quality of life is the foundation that informs person-centred support and is the primary criterion in the evaluation of this support.

We hope that this book serves as a guide in the application of this unified framework and that it leads to improvements in the service design and delivery for people with intellectual disabilities. More importantly, though, that it leads to improvements in the individual's quality of life by delivering more personalised supports.

 Enabling Capable Environments © Pavilion Publishing and Media Ltd and its licensors 2024.

Resources

Appendix One: Capable Environments Periodic Service Review (PSR) Sheet (ten a day)

(Outlined in Hume *et al*, 2021

Standard 1: Positive social interactions	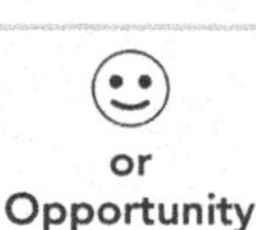 or Opportunity

Standard 2: Support for communication	☺ or Opportunity

Standard 3: Participation in meaningful activity	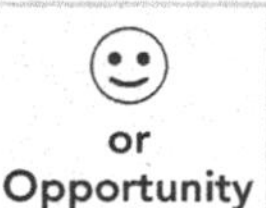 or Opportunity

Standard 4: Consistent and predictable environments	☺ or Opportunity

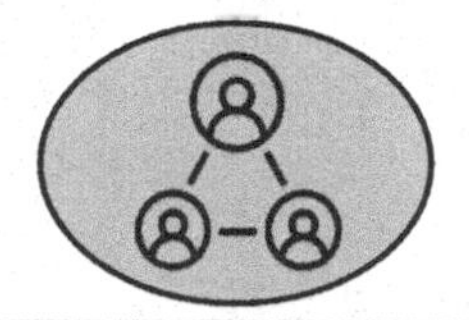

Standard 5: Establish and maintain relationships.	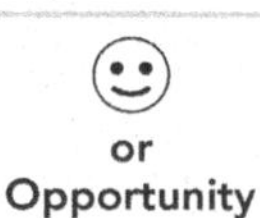 or Opportunity

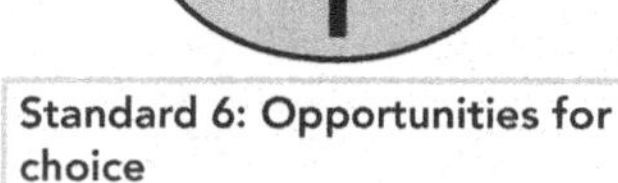

Standard 6: Opportunities for choice	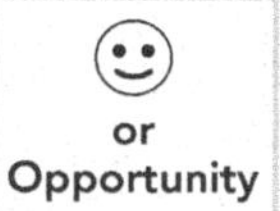 or Opportunity

Standard 7: Independent functioning	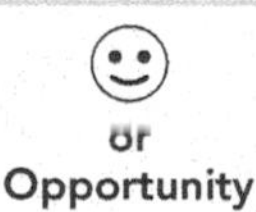 or Opportunity

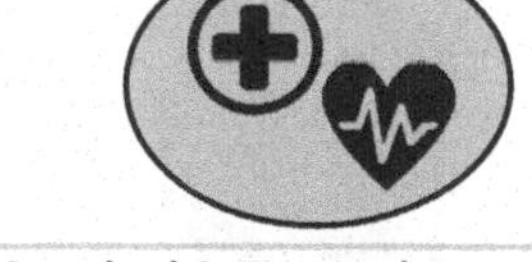

Standard 8: Personal care and health	 or Opportunity

Standard 9: Physical environment	☺ or Opportunity

Standard 10: Mindful skilled carers	☺ or Opportunity

Appendix Two: Capable Environments Appraisal Tool

Characteristic	What does this involve?	Why is this important?	Evidence	
			Working well	***Opportunity to develop***
Positive social interactions	Carers like the person and interact (speak, sign, physically etc.) frequently with them in ways that the person enjoys and understands.	In situations where the person receives unconditional, positive social interactions, they are less likely to display challenging behaviour to obtain social interaction. Carers who establish good relationships with individuals can embed any necessary less positive interactions (e.g. physical care that may be uncomfortable or distressing). Most people (with and without learning disabilities) want to receive positive social interactions from those around them.		

Support for communication	Carers communicate in ways the person understands. They are able to notice, interpret and respond to the person's own communications, whether indicated by speech, sign, gesture, behaviour or other. This support for communication is seen across all areas of the person's life and people are supported in rich communication environments. This knowledge of communication is shared across environments and with unfamiliar communication partners (e.g. through the use of communication passports).	Challenging behaviour is less likely when the person understands and is understood by those around them. Most people (with and without learning disabilities) want to communicate with those around them, especially those they are close to.		

Enabling Capable Environments © Pavilion Publishing and Media Ltd and its licensors 2024.

Support for participation in meaningful activity	Carers provide tailored assistance for the individual to engage meaningfully in preferred domestic, leisure, work activities and social interactions. Assistance meaningfully employs speech, manual signs, symbols or objects of reference as appropriate.	Challenging behaviour is less likely when the person is meaningfully occupied. Skilled support ensures that they can participate at least partially even in relatively complex activities so that they learn to cope with demands and difficulties that might otherwise provoke challenging behaviour. Most people (with and without learning disabilities) like to be busy.		
Provision of consistent and predictable environments that honour personalised routines and activities	Carers support the person consistently so that the person's experience is similar no matter who is providing the support. Carers use a range of communication and other approaches tailored to the individual (e.g. visual timetables, regular routines) to ensure that the person understands as much as possible about what is happening and what is about to happen.	Challenging behaviour is more likely when the person is supported inconsistently or when in transition between one activity/environment and another. Most people (with and without learning disabilities) value consistent and predictable support.		

Enabling Capable Environments © Pavilion Publishing and Media Ltd and its licensors 2024.

Support to establish and/ or maintain relationships with family and friends	Carers understand the lifelong importance to most people of their families, and the significance of relationships with others (partners, friends, acquaintances etc.). Carers actively support all such relationships while being aware of the risks that sometimes arise in close or intimate relationships.	Challenging behaviour is less likely when the person is with family members or others with whom they have positive relationships. For most people (with and without learning disabilities), relationships with family and friends are a central part of their life.		
Provision of opportunities for choice	Carers ensure that the individual is involved as much as possible in deciding how to spend their time and the nature of the support they receive from the relatively mundane (e.g. choice of breakfast cereal) to the more serious (e.g. who supports them).	Challenging behaviour is less likely when the person is doing things that they have chosen to do or with people that they have chosen to be with. Most people (with and without learning disabilities) value the opportunity to decide things for themselves.		

Enabling Capable Environments © Pavilion Publishing and Media Ltd and its licensors 2024.

Encouragement of more independent functioning	Carers support the individual to learn new skills, to try new experiences and to take more responsibility for their own occupation, care and safety.	The development of new skills and independent functioning enables the individual to have more control over their life. Most people (with and without learning disabilities) like to be independent.		
Personal care and health support	Carers are attentive to the individual's personal and healthcare needs, identifying pain/discomfort, enabling access to professional healthcare support where necessary and tactfully supporting compliance with healthcare treatments.	Challenging behaviour is less likely when the individual is healthy and not in pain or discomfort. Most people (with and without learning disabilities) attach the highest possible value to "good health" and want to receive personal support in dignified ways.		

Provision of acceptable physical environment	Carers support the individual to access and maintain environments which meet the individual's needs/preferences in respect of space, aesthetics (including sensory preferences), noise, lighting, state of repair and safety.	Challenging behaviour is less likely in the absence of environmental 'pollutants' (e.g. excessive noise). Most people (with and without learning disabilities) want to live and work in safe, attractive environments where they feel at home.		
Mindful, skilled carers	Carers understand both the general causes of challenging behaviour and the specific influences on the individual's behaviour. They draw on the expert knowledge of the individual's family and friends to improve their understanding. They reflect on, and adjust, their support to prevent and/or quickly identify circumstances that may provoke challenging behaviour.	Challenging behaviour is less likely when carers understand its causes and do not take it as personally directed at them. Most people (with and without learning disabilities), when in situations where they require support, want their carers to attend to and know what they are doing.		

Enabling Capable Environments © Pavilion Publishing and Media Ltd and its licensors 2024.

Effective management and support	Carers are managed and/or supported by individuals with administrative competence and the skills to lead all aspects of capable practice.	Challenging behaviour is less likely when carers are well-managed, led and supported. Most people (with and without learning disabilities) want to be confident that their carers (if they need them) are, themselves, well supported and can get help when they need it.		
Effective organisational context	Support provided by carers is delivered and arranged within a broader understanding of challenging behaviour that recognises (among other things) the need to ensure safety and quality of care for both individuals and carers.	Challenging behaviour is less likely when positive behaviour support informs the culture of families, service providers and service commissioners. Most people (with and without learning disabilities) want to receive evidence-based, well-governed supports.		

Adapted from McGill *et al* (2020)
Outlined in Hume *et al* (2021)

Enabling Capable Environments © Pavilion Publishing and Media Ltd and its licensors 2024.

Appendix Three: Practice Leadership Mentoring & Observation Guide

Celebrating success and identifying opportunities: (adapted from Beadle-Brown *et al.*, 2015).

> *"Tell me, and I will listen; Teach me, and I'll remember; Involve me, and I will learn."*
> – Benjamin Franklin

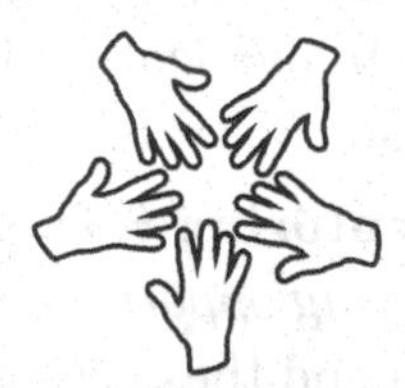

The original practice leadership observation guide by Beadle-Brown *et al.*, 2015 was developed in the context of research of service development/evaluation. In their *Observational Practice Leadership Measure* there are five domains:

1. Allocating and organising staff to deliver support how and when it is needed.
2. ***Coaching staff to deliver better support by watching how staff support people and collaboratively identifying what is working well and what can be improved.***
3. Reviewing the quality of support as part of individual supervision.
4. Reviewing how well teams work in enabling people to engage in meaningful activities and relationships as part of team meetings.
5. The manager focuses all aspects of their work on the continuous improvement of quality of life and how well staff support this.

Our guide provides a mentorship support guide (exemplar) to coach practice leaders in domain two:

Coaching staff to deliver better support
We have adapted this guide to fit with a **collaborative approach to mentoring** practice leaders. This guide is designed to be used by practice leaders and their mentors (mentors can be a parent, a teacher, someone who provides supervision in practice etc), the key factor is that the person in the mentorship role is proficient in supporting the practice leader in identifying what is working well in how teams provide someone's support and what can be improved.

Some key points to consider about this guide:

- It is not an audit or score sheet.
- It is a tool to collaboratively identify good practice and build on this.
- It is a tool to collaboratively identify the barriers to good practice and look at resolutions to these barriers.
- We recommend as a minimum, readers are familiar with the contents of chapters 5, 6 & 7 within this book 'Enabling Capable Environments Using Practice Leadership: A Unique Framework for Supporting People with Intellectual Disabilities and Their Carers'. In particular the scaffolding approach section of chapter 5 before using this guide.
- Our **Practice Leadership Mentoring & Observation Guide** is focussed on *Celebrating success and identifying opportunities*; therefore it also identifies what is working and how to expand these positive good practices.

A key focus of a practice leader is to help move people from being able to say what needs to be done (verbal competence) to a place where they can mentor others in providing good quality supports, in practice (practice competence) where people do what is needed (Chapter 5)

In chapter 5 we discuss how a form of scaffolding, from knowing to doing fits with many of the components of practice leadership as outlined above. Typically, teams need support to move from reading a support plan, teams need time to be spent with them, with the practice lead providing clarifying, coaching, and providing feedback at each of the steps illustrated below.

Figure One: Scaffolding support plan competency (Five tiers to competency)

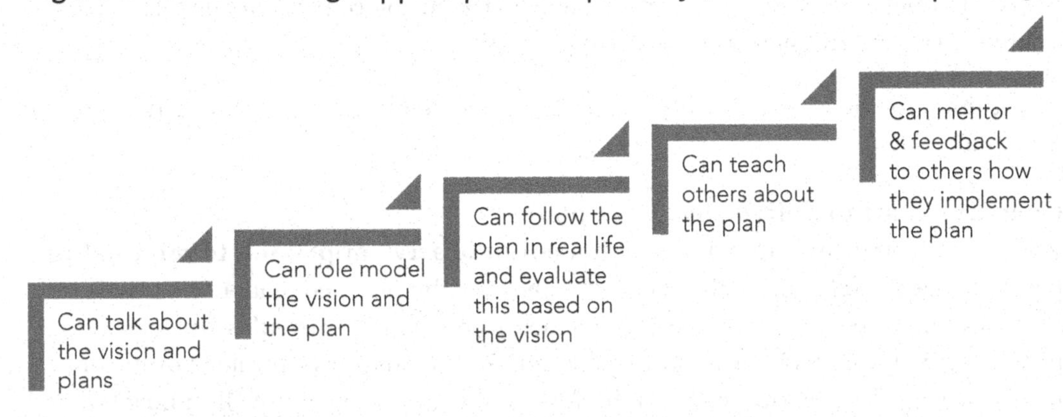

(Hume *et al*., 2024)

Enabling Capable Environments © Pavilion Publishing and Media Ltd and its licensors 2024.

In chapter 6 we identify that practice leadership involves **co-producing a shared vision** of a successful service and supports. The practice leaders must:

- **Focus** on all aspects of service delivery, the individual's quality of life, and how the team support this.
- **Allocate** and organise support to deliver on the shared vision when and how the individual wants/needs this.
- **Coach** and mentor good practice and provide feedback.
- **Review** the quality of support as outlined in the vision by means of a continuous improvement cycle.

Our Practice Leadership Mentoring & Observation Guide (table 1 below) combines the scaffolding approach and the four key elements of practice leadership guiding practice leaders.

To use this guide, you should:

- Ask a mentor to observe your practice using the guide below a couple of times in a week, even just for 20 minutes and use the guide below to identify what is working well, what can be improved and what actions and support is needed to bring about positive changes in practice.
- As the mentor briefly outline what the core activity of the practice leader was during you time observing *(Row 1)*
- As you observe consider which current practice rating applies based on the information in *What it looked like section (Column 1 & 2)*
- Following the observation time as a mentor spend time discussing with the practice leader what elements were working well *(Column 3)* What could be improved *(Column 4)* and agree an action mentorship plan about how improvements can be made and how success can be shared *(Column 5)*.

Table One: Practice Leadership Mentoring & Observation Guide : Celebrating success and identifying opportunities:

The context of this guide is to mentor, coach, and support people into practice leadership roles and to sustain people in these roles.

Row 1 Activity observed.				
Column 1 Current practices rating	Column 2 What it looked like	Column 3 What is working well?	Column 4 What could be improved (be specific on how it can be improved)	Column 5 Actions & mentorship plan (what do you need to do and what support can your mentor provide)
1	No opportunity or observation that the practice leader spends any time coaching or modelling. He/she is rarely of the office and when on shift works alone. Staff are doing things that they shouldn't be doing, and practice leader is not noticing or is noticing, commenting on this to others but not giving feedback to staff.			
2	The practice leader spends some time informally watching staff but does not use that information to try to develop staff practices. Their own practice where observed is ok but they don't direct or support other staff. There is no evidence that they model or coach staff in any way, even on an adhoc basis.			

Enabling Capable Environments © Pavilion Publishing and Media Ltd and its licensors 2024.

3	The practice leader does not spend time formally observing but can give examples of how they have spotted things while walking about or working in the same area as other staff and then used that information to give feedback to staff, feed into supervision etc. Their practice is quite good, but they can't give good examples of how they have modelled these skills for a particular staff or activity.			
4	The practice leader spends some time in formal observation and giving feedback and is seen to provide modelling or coaching (or gives a good account of how he/she has done this). However, opportunities for this are left somewhat to chance and there is no system in place where manager/supervisor spends time regularly with each member of staff. So, who receives modelling will depend on who the manager is on shift with.			

Enabling Capable Environments © Pavilion Publishing and Media Ltd and its licensors 2024.

5	You observe or the practice leader gives examples of how he/she regularly observes and works with staff. There is a system of some sort in place to ensure that all staff are observed and receive feedback on a regular basis and the leader can give good examples of how he/she has done this. Examples shows that they are focusing on active support.			

Other detailed guides to observation of practice can be found on the United Response website: What does good look like? Available at https://www.unitedresponse.org.uk/resource/what-does-good-look-like/

Enabling Capable Environments © Pavilion Publishing and Media Ltd and its licensors 2024.

References

Abawi, L.A. (2015) 'Inclusion 'from the gate in': wrapping students with personalised learning support', *International Journal of Pedagogies and Learning*, 10(1), pp. 47-61. Available at: DOI: 10.1080/22040552.2015.1084676

Ahmed, M. (2007) *Interview with Jim Mansell*. Available at: https://www.communitycare.co.uk/2007/11/12/interview-with-jim-mansell/ (Accessed: 22 November 2023).

Allen, D., McGill, P., Hastings, R., Toogood, S., Baker, P., Gore, N. and Hughes, J.C. (2013) 'Implementing positive behavioural support: changing social and organisational contexts', *International Journal of Positive Behavioural Support*, 3(2), pp. 32-41. Available at: https://hcpbs.org/wp-content/uploads/2018/06/implementing-pbs-in-social-organizational-contexts.pdf

Aranzamendez, G., James, D. and Toms, R. (2015), Psychological Safety. *Nursing Forum*, 50: 171-178. https://doi.org/10.1111/nuf.12084

Atkins, P.W.B. and Parker, S.K. (2012) in Bailey, S., and West, M. (2022) *What is Compassionate Leadership?* Available at: https://www.kingsfund.org.uk/publications/what-is-compassionate-leadership (Accessed: 4 January 2024).

Bailey, S. and West, M. (2022) *What is Compassionate Leadership?* Available at: https://www.kingsfund.org.uk/publications/what-is-compassionate-leadership (Accessed: 4 January 2024).

Baker, P., Appleton, P. and Williams, R. (2017) 'An examination of the addition of video-informed reflective practice to the active support toolkit', *British Journal of Learning Disabilities*, 45(17), pp. 180-189. Available at: https://doi.org/10.1111/bld.12193

Baker P. A. (2000) 'Measurement of community participation and use of leisure by service users with intellectual disabilities: The Guernsey Community Participation and Leisure Assessment (GCPLA)', *Journal of Applied Research in Intellectual Disabilities*, 13(3), pp. 169–185. Available at: https://doi.org/10.1046/j.1468-3148.2000.00015.x

BBC Panorama (2011) Undercover Care: The Abuse Exposed. www.bbc.co.uk/programmes/b011pwt6 (Accessed 29 February 2024).

BBC Panorama (2019) Undercover Hospital Abuse Scandal. www.bbc.co.uk/programmes/m00059qb (Accessed 29 February 2024).

BBC News. (2020) 'Muckamore Abbey Hospital: Timeline of Abuse Allegations', *BBC News*, 7 September. Available at: www.bbc.co.uk/news/ uk-northern-ireland-49498971 (Accessed 4 October 2023).

Beach Centre on Disabilities (2006) *Family quality of life scale*. Lawrence, KS: Author.

Beail, N., Frankish, P. and Skelly, A. (2021) *Trauma and Intellectual Disability*. Shoreham-by-Sea: Pavilion Publishing & Media.

Beadle-Brown, J., Bigby, C., & Bould, E. (2015) 'Observing practice leadership in intellectual and developmental disability services', *Journal of Intellectual Disability Research*, 59(12), pp. 1081-1093. Available at: DOI: 10.1111/jir.12208

Beadle-Brown, J., Mansell, J., Ashman, B., Ockenden, J., Iles, R. and Whelton, B. (2014) 'Practice leadership and active support in residential services for people with intellectual disabilities: an exploratory study', *Journal of Intellectual Disability Research*, 58(9), pp. 838-50. Available at: DOI: 10.1111/jir.12099

Beadle-Brown., and Murphy, B. (2016) *What does good look like? A guide for observing in services for people with learning disabilities and/or autism*. United Response and Tizard Centre.

Beadle-Brown, J., Murphy, B. and Bradshaw, J. (2017) *Person-centred active support*. 2nd edn. Shoreham-by-Sea: Pavilion Publishing & Media.

Bigby, C., Anderson, S. and Cameron, N. (2018) 'Identifying conceptualizations and theories of change embedded in interventions to facilitate community participation for people with intellectual disability: A scoping review', *Journal of Applied Research in Intellectual Disabilities*, 31(2), pp. 165-180. Available at: doi: 10.1111/jar.12390. dd

Bigby, C. and Beadle-Brown, J. (2016) 'Improving Quality of Life Outcomes in Supported Accommodation for People with Intellectual Disability: What Makes a Difference?', *Journal of Applied Research in Intellectual Disabilities*, 31(2), pp. 182-200. Available at: doi: 10.1111/jar.12291

Bigby, C. and Bould, E. (2017) 'Guide to Good Group Homes, Evidence about what makes the most difference to the quality of group homes'. *Centre for Applied Disability Research*. Available at: www.cadr.org.au

Bigby, C. and Beadle-Brown, J. (2018) 'Improving Quality of Life Outcomes in Supported Accommodation for People with Intellectual Disability: What Makes a Difference?', *Journal of Applied Research in Intellectual Disability*, 31(2), pp. 182-200. Available at: doi: 10.1111/jar.12291.

Bigby, C., Clement, T., Mansell, J. and Beadle-Brown, J. (2009) "It's pretty hard with our ones, they can't talk, the more able bodied can participate': staff attitudes about the applicability of disability policies to people with severe and profound intellectual disabilities', *Journal of Intellectual Disabilities Research*, 53(4), pp. 363-76. Available at: doi: 10.1111/j.1365-2788.2009.01154.x.

Bloom, S.L. (1995) 'Creating sanctuary in the school', *Journal for a Just and Caring Education*, 1(4), pp. 403–33. Available at: https://sandrabloom.com/wp-content/uploads/1995-Bloom-Creating-Sanctuary-in-the-School.pdf

Bould, E., Beadle-Brown, J., Bigby, C. and Lacono, T. (2018) 'The role of practice leadership in active support: impact of practice leaders' presence in supported accommodation services', *International Journal of Developmental Disabilities*, 64(2), pp. 75-80. Available at: DOI: 10.1080/20473869.2016.1229524

Bowring, D.L., Totsika, V., Hastings, R.P., Toogood, S. and Griffith, G.M. (2017) 'Challenging behaviours in adults with an intellectual disability: A total population study and exploration of risk indices', *British Journal of Clinical Psychology*, 56(1), 16–32. Available at: DOI: 10.1111/bjc.12118

Bowring, D. L., Painter, J. and Hastings, R. P. (2019) 'Prevalence of Challenging Behaviour in Adults with Intellectual Disabilities, Correlates, and Association with Mental Health', *Current Developmental Disorders Reports*, 6(4), pp. 173–181. Available at: doi: 10.1007/s40474-019-00175-9.

Bundy, A.C., Lane, S.J. and Murray, E.A. (Eds.) (2002) *Sensory integration: Theory and practice* (2nd ed). Philadelphia: F. A. Davis Company.

 Enabling Capable Environments © Pavilion Publishing and Media Ltd and its licensors 2024.

Buntinx, W.H.E. (2015) 'Understanding Disability: A Strengths-based Approach', in M.L. Wehmeyer (Ed.), *The oxford handbook of positive psychology and disability*. New York: Oxford University Press, pp. 7-18.

Caldwell, P. (2012) *Delicious Conversations: Reflections on autism, intimacy and communication*. Shoreham-by-Sea: Pavilion Publishing & Media.

Capie, A. (1996) 'The essential elements in effective evaluation', in R. McConkey (Ed.), *Innovations in evaluating services for people with intellectual disabilities*. Chorley: Lisieux Hall Publications, pp. 73-90.

Care Quality Commission (2022) *Right Support, Right Care, Right Culture: How CQC Regulates Providers Supporting Autistic People and People with a Learning Disability (updated 2022)*. Available at: https://www.cqc.org.uk/sites/default/files/2022-06/900582%20Right%20support%20right%20care%20right%20culture_v5_0.pdf

Carr, E.G., Horner, R.H., Turnbull, A.P., Marquis, J.G., McLaughlin, D.M., McAtee, M.L., Smith, C.E., Ryan, K.A., Ruef, M.B., Doolabh, A. and Braddock, D. (Eds.) (1999) *Positive Behavior Support for People with Developmental Disabilities: A Research Synthesis*, Washington: American Association on Mental Retardation.

Carr, E. G., Dunlap, G., Horner, R. H., Koegel, R. L., Turnbull, A. P., Sailor, W., ... and Fox, L. (2002) 'Positive behavior support: Evolution of an applied science', *Journal of positive behavior interventions*, **4**(1), pp. 4-16. Available at: https://doi.org/10.1177/10983007020040010

Carlsson, Õ.U. and Adolfsson, P. (2022) 'No ordinary adult life: Living conditions from the perspective of adults with intellectual disabilities', *Journal of Intellectual Disabilities*, **0**(0), pp. 1-20. Available at: https://journals.sagepub.com/doi/pdf/10.1177/17446295221107284

Carr, E.G. (1996) The transfiguration of behavior analysis: Strategies for survival. *Journal of Behavioral Education*, 6, 263—270.

Carr, E.G., Levin, L., McConnachie, G., Carlson, J.I., Kemp, D.C. & Smith, C. E. (1994) *Communication-based intervention for problem behavior: A user's guide for producing positive change*. Baltimore: Paul H Brookes Publishing.

Causton, J., Tracy-Bronson, C.P., and MacLeod, K. (2015) 'Beyond treats and timeouts: Humanistic behavior supports in inclusive classrooms', *International Journal of Whole Schooling*, **11**(1), pp. 68-84. Available at: https://doi.org/10.1177/109830070200400102

Conder, J.A. and Mirfin-Veitch, B.F. (2020) '"Getting by": People with learning disability and the financial responsibility of independent living', *British Journal of Learning Disabilities*, **48**(3), pp. 251-257. Available at: https://doi.org/10.1111/bld.12329

Crates, N. and Spicer, M. (2016) 'Reactive strategies within a positive behavioural support framework for reducing the episodic severity of aggression', *International Journal of Positive Behavioural Support*, **6**(1), pp. 24–34. Available at: https://www.ingentaconnect.com/content/bild/ijpbs/2016/00000006/00000001/art00004

Department of Health (2001) Valuing People: A New Strategy for Learning Disability for the 21st Century. Cm. 5086. London: Department of Health.

Department of Health (2009) *Valuing People Now: A new three-year strategy for people with learning disabilities*. London: HMSO.

Department of Health (2012) *Transforming care: A national response to Winterbourne View Hospital: Department of Health Review Final Report*. Available at: https://assets.publishing.service.gov.uk/media/5a7b91f7ed915d13110601c3/final-report.pdf

Donnellan, A. M., Hill, D.A. and Leary, M.R. (2012) 'Rethinking autism: Implications of sensory and movement differences for understanding and support', *Frontiers in Integrative Neuroscience*, **6**(124), pp. 1-11. Available at: https://doi.org/10.3389/fnint.2012.00124

Donnellan, A.M., LaVigna, G., Negri-Shoultz, N. and Fassbender, L. (1988) *Progress without punishment: Effective approaches for learners with behavior problems*. Columbia University: Teachers College Press.

Doody, C. (2009) 'Multi-element behaviour support as a model for the delivery of a human rights based approach for working with people with intellectual disabilities and behaviours that challenge', *British Journal of Learning Disabilities*, **37**(4), pp. 293–299. Available at: DOI:10.1111/j.1468-3156.2009.00585.x

Durand, V. M. and Crimmins, D. B. (1992) *The Motivation Assessment Scale (MAS) administration guide*. Topeka, KS: Monaco and Associates.

Edmondson, A. C. (1999) Psychological safety and learning behavior in work teams, *Administrative Science Quarterly*, **44**(2), pp. 350–383. Available at: https://doi.org/10.2307/2666999

Edmondson, A. C. (2004) 'Psychological safety, trust, and learning in organizations: A group-level lens', in R. Kramer and K. Cook (Eds.), *Trust in organizations: Dilemmas and approaches*. New York: Russell Sage Foundation, pp. 239–272.

Emerson, E., Felce, D., McGill, P. and Mansell, J. (1994) 'Introduction', in E. Emerson, P. McGill, and J. Mansell (Eds.), *Severe Learning Disabilities and Challenging Behaviours. Designing High Quality Services*. Hong Kong: Springer Science Business Media Dordrecht, pp. 11-22.

Emerson, E. and Bromley, J. (1995) 'The form and function of challenging behaviours', *Journal of Intellectual Disability Research*, **39**(5), 388–398

Emerson, E. and Enfield, S. (2011) *Challenging Behaviour*. 3rd edn. Cambridge: Cambridge University Press.

Emerson, E., Fortune, N., Llewellyn, G. and Stancliffe, R. (2021) 'Loneliness, social support, social isolation and wellbeing among working age adults with and without disability: Cross-sectional study', *Disability and Health Journal*, **14**(1), pp. 1-7. Available at: https://doi.org/10.1016/j.dhjo.2020.100965.

Emerson, E., Hastings, R. and McGill (1994) 'Values, attitudes and service ideology', in E. Emerson, P. McGill, and J. Mansell (Eds.), *Severe Learning Disabilities and Challenging Behaviours. Designing High Quality Services*. Hong Kong: Springer Science Business Media Dordrecht, pp. 155-172.

Emerson, E. and Hatton, C. (2014) *Health inequalities and people with intellectual disabilities*. Cambridge: Cambridge University Press.

Emerson, E., McGill, P. and Mansell, J. (Eds) (1994) *Severe Learning Disabilities and Challenging Behaviours. Designing High Quality Services*. Hong Kong: Springer Science Business Media Dordrecht.

Ginott, H.G. (1993) *Teacher and child: A book for parents and teachers*. Prentice Hall & IBD

Gore, N.J., McGill, P., Toogood, S., Allen, D., Hughes, J.C., Baker, P., Hastings, R.P., Noone, S.J. and Denne, L.D. (2013). 'Definition and scope for positive behavioural support', *International Journal of Positive Behavioural Support*, **3**(2), pp. 14-23.

 Enabling Capable Environments © Pavilion Publishing and Media Ltd and its licensors 2024.

Gore, N. J. *et al*. (2022) 'Positive behavioural support in the UK: A state of the nation report', *International Journal of Positive Behvioural Support*, **12**(1), pp. 1–44. Available at: https://www.ingentaconnect.com/contentone/bild/ijpbs/2022/00000012/a00101s1/art00001.

Grey, I.M. and Hastings, R. (2005) 'Evidence based practice in the treatment of behaviour disorders in intellectual disability', *Current Opinion in Psychiatry*, **18**(5), pp. 469–475. Available at: DOI: 10.1097/01.yco.0000179482.54767.cf

Grey, I.M. and McClean, B. (2007) 'Service User Outcomes of Staff Training in Positive Behaviour Support Using Person-Focused Training: A Control Group Study', *Journal of Applied Research in Intellectual Disabilities*, **20**(1), pp. 6–15. Available at: https://doi.org/10.1111/j.1468-3148.2006.00335.x

Harding, C. (2021) 'Providing emotionally aware care in the positive behavioural support framework', in N. Beail., P. Frankish. and A. Skelly. (Eds.), *Trauma and Intellectual Disability*. Shoreham-by-Sea: Pavilion Publishing & Media, pp.103-119.

Hastings R. P., Allen D., Baker P., Gore N. J., Hughes J. C., McGill P. et al. (2013) 'A conceptual framework for understanding why challenging behaviours occur in people with developmental disabilities', *International Journal of Positive Behavioural Support* **3**(2), pp. 5–13. Available at: https://pbsnec.co.uk/wp-content/uploads/2021/10/Hastings-et-al-a-conceptual-framework.pdf

Heller, T. (2002) 'Residential settings and outcomes for individuals with intellectual disabilities', *Current Opinion in Psychiatry,* **15**(5), pp. 1-6. Available at: DOI: 10.1097/00001504-200209000-00007

Horner, R. H. et al. (1990) 'Towards a technology of ' nonaversive Toward a Technology of " Nonaversive " Behavioral Support', *Journal of the Association for Persons with Severe Handicaps.*, **15**(3), pp. 125–132. Available at: doi:10.1177/154079699001500301.

Horner, R.H., Sugai, G. and Anderson, C.M. (2010) 'Examining the Evidence Base for School-Wide Positive Behavior Support', *Focus on Exceptional Children*, **42**(8): pp.1-14. Available at: DOI: 10.17161/fec.v42i8.6906

Howell, R. W., and Vetter, H. J. (1976) *Language in behavior*. New York, Human Sciences Press.

Hughes, E.C, Venegas, S., LaVigna, G.W. and Willis, T.J. (2014) 'Effective practices for children with challenging behaviour: using positive behaviour support', in M. Lovell and O. Udwin (Eds), *Intellectual Disabilities and Challenging Behaviour.* United Kingdom: Association for Child and Adolescent Mental Health (ACAMH), pp. 79–88.

Human Rights Act (1998): Elizabeth ll. Chapter 42. (1998). London: The Stationery Office.

Hume, L., Khan, N. and Reilly, M. (2021) 'Building capable environments using practice leadership', *Tizard Learning Disability Review*, **26**(1), pp. 1–8. Available at: doi: 10.1108/TLDR-07-2020-0017.

Hume, L., Delrée, J., and McMeel, A. (2023) Challenging and distressed behaviour in people with intellectual disabilities, the role of intellectual disability nurses. in Mafuba (Ed), Learning and Intellectual Disability Nursing Practice, pp.273-298. Routledge.

Johnstone L, Boyle M, Cromby J, *et al*. (2018) *The Power Threat Meaning Framework: Towards the Identification of Patterns in Emotional Distress, Unusual Experiences and Troubled or Troubling Behaviour, as an Alternative to Functional Psychiatric Diagnosis*. UK: British Psychological Society

Johnstone L, Dallos R (eds) (2006) *Formulation in Psychology and Psychotherapy: Making Sense of People's Problems*. East Sussex: Routledge.

Johnson, H., Douglas, J., Bigby, C. and Iacono, T. (2012) 'Social interaction with adults with severe intellectual disability: Having fun and hanging out', *Journal of Applied Research in Intellectual Disabilities*, **25**(4), pp. 329–341. Available at: https://doi.org/10.1111/j.1468-3148.2011.00669.x

Kotter, J. P. (1996) *Leading Change*. Boston: Harvard Business School Press.

Kuypers, L. M. (2011) *The zones of regulation: A curriculum designed to foster self-regulation and emotional control*. Santa Clara, CA: Think Social Publishing.

Laal, M. and Laal, M. (2012) 'Collaborative learning: What is it?', *Procedia – Social and Behavioral Sciences*, **31**, pp. 491-495. Available at: https://doi.org/10.1016/j.sbspro.2011.12.092

LaVigna, G.W., Hughes, E.C., Potter, G., Spicer, M., Hume, L., Willis, T.J. and Huerta, E. (2022) 'Needed independent and dependent variables in multi-element behavior support plans addressing severe behavior problems', *Perspectives on Behavior Science*, **45**(2), pp. 421–444. Available at: DOI: 10.1007/s40614-022-00331-4

La Vigna G. and Willis T. (1996) 'A model of non-aversive behavioural support', *Positive Practices*, **111**(4), pp. 1–24. Available at : https://hcpbs.org/wp-content/uploads/2018/08/antecedent-analyses.pdf

LaVigna, G. and Willis, T. (2005) 'A Positive Behavioural Support Model for Breaking the Barriers to Social and Community Inclusion', *Learning Disability Review*, **10** (2), pp. 16–23. Available at: https://doi.org/10.1108/13595474200500016

LaVigna, G. W. and Willis, T. J. (2012) 'The efficacy of positive behavioural support with the most challenging behaviour: The evidence and its implications', *Journal of Intellectual and Developmental Disability*, **37**(3), pp. 185–195. Availbale at: doi: 10.3109/13668250.2012.696597.

LaVigna, G., Willis, T.J., Shaull, J.F., Abedi, M. and Sweitzer, M. (1994) *The Periodic Service Review: A Total Quality Assurance System for Human Services and Education*. Baltimore: Brookes Publishing.

Learning Disabilities Mortality Review (LeDeR) Programme (2021) *Annual Report 2020*. Available at: https://www.england.nhs.uk/wp-content/uploads/2021/06/LeDeR-bristol-annual-report-2020.pdf

Lovett, H. (1996) *Learning to Listen: Positive Approaches and People with Difficult Behavior*. Baltimore: Brookes Publishing.

Mansell, J. (2007) *Services for people with learning disabilities and challenging behaviour or mental health needs, Services for people with learning disabilities and challenging behaviour or Mental Health needs* (Revised Edition). London: Department of Health.

Mansell, J. and Beadle-Brown, J. (2004) 'Person-centred planning or person-centred action? Policy and practice in intellectual disability services', *Journal of Applied Research in Intellectual Disabilities*,**17**(1) pp. 1–9. Available at: https://doi.org/10.1111/j.1468-3148.2004.00175.x

Mansell, J. and Beadle-Brown, J. (2012) *Active support: enabling and empowering people with intellectual disabilities*. London: Jessica Kingsley Publishers.

Mansell, J., Beadle-Brown, J., Ashman, B. and Ockenden, J. (2004) *Person-centred active support: A multi-media training resource for staff to enable participation, inclusion and choice for people with learning disabilities*. Shoreham-by-Sea: Pavilion Publishing & Media.

Mansell, J., Beadle-Brown, J., Whelton, B., Beckett, C. & Hutchinson, A. (2008) 'Effect of Service Structure and Organization on Staff Care Practices in Small Community Homes for People with

 Enabling Capable Environments © Pavilion Publishing and Media Ltd and its licensors 2024.

Intellectual Disabilities', *Journal of Applied Research in Intellectual Disabilities*, **21**(5), pp. 398-413. Available at: https://doi.org/10.1111/j.1468-3148.2007.00410

Mansell, J., Elliott, T.E. and Beadle-Brown, J. (2005) *Active Support Measure (Revised)*. Canterbury, UK: Tizard Centre.

Mansell, J., Felce, D., Jenkins, J., de Kock, U. and Toogood, A. (1983) 'A Wessex home from home: a staffed house for mentally handicapped adults'. *Nursing Times* **79**(31), pp. 51-3, 56. Available at: PMID: 6554684.

Mansell, J., Felce, D., Jenkins, J., de Kock, U. and Toogood, A. (1987) *Developing staffed housing for people with mental handicaps*. Tunbridge Wells: Costello.

Mansell, J., Hughes. H. and McGill. P. (1994) 'Maintaining local residential placements', in E. Emerson, P. McGill, and J. Mansell (Eds.), *Severe Learning Disabilities and Challenging Behaviours. Designing High Quality Services*. Hong Kong: Springer Science Business Media Dordrecht, pp. 190-205.

Matson J.L. and Vollmer T.R. (1995) *The Questions about Behavioral Function (QABF) user's guide*. Baton Rouge, LA: Scientific Publishers.

McClean, B., Dench, C., Grey, I., Shanahan, S., Fitzsimons, E., Hendler, J., and Corrigan, M. (2005) 'Person focused training: A model for delivering positive behavioural supports to people with challenging behaviours', *Journal of Intellectual Disability*, **49**(5), pp. 340-352. Available at: DOI: 10.1111/j.1365-2788.2005.00669.x

McClean, B. and Grey, I. (2012a) 'A component analysis of positive behaviour support plans', *Journal of Intellectual and Developmental Disability*, **37**(3), pp. 221-231. Available at: doi: 10.3109/13668250.2012.704981.

McClean, B. and Grey, I. (2012b) 'An Evaluation of an Intervention Sequence Outline in Positive Behaviour Support for People with Autism and Severe Escape-Motivated Challenging Behaviour', *Journal of Intellectual Disability*, **37**(3), pp. 209-220. Available at: DOI: 10.3109/13668250.2012.704982

McGill, P. Bradshaw, J. Smyth, G. Hurman, M. and Roy, A. (2014) *Capable environments*. Available at: www.kcl.ac.uk/sspp/policy-institute/scwru/news/

McGill, P., Vanono, L., Clover, W., Smyth, E., Cooper, V., Hopkins, L., Barratt, N., Joyce, C., Henderson, K., Sekasi, S., Davis, S., & Deveau, R. (2018) Reducing challenging behaviour of adults with intellectual disabilities in supported accommodation: A cluster randomized controlled trial of setting-wide positive behaviour support. *Research in developmental disabilities*, **81**, pp.143–154. https://doi.org/10.1016/j.ridd.2018.04.020

McGill, P., Bradshaw, J., Smyth, G., Hurman, M. and Roy, A. (2020) 'Capable environments, *Tizard Learning Disability Review*, **25**(3), pp. 109-116. Available at: 116. https://kar.kent.ac.uk/83154/1/PDF_Proof.PDF

McGill, P. and Toogood, S. (1994) *'Organising community placements Severe Learning Disabilities and Challenging Behaviours'*, in E. Emerson, P. McGill, and J. Mansell (Eds.), *Severe Learning Disabilities and Challenging Behaviours. Designing High Quality Services*. Hong Kong: Springer Science Business Media Dordrecht, pp. 173-189.

McKim, J. (2021). *Active Support and "meaningful activity." What is the meaning of "meaningful"*. Available at: https://oxfordhealth-nhs.archive.knowledgearc.net/handle/123456789/942

McLaughlin, TW, Denney, MK, Snyder, PA and Welsh, JL (2012) 'Behaviour support interventions implemented by families of young children: Examination of contextual fit', *Journal of Positive Behaviour Interventions*, **14**(2), pp. 87-97. Available at: https://doi.org/10.1177/1098300711411305

MENCAP (2007) *Death by Indifference: Following up the Treat me right! report*. Available at: https://www.mencap.org.uk/sites/default/files/2016-07/DBIreport.pdf

Mithen, J., Aitken, Z., Ziersch, A. and Kavanagh, A.M. (2015) 'Inequalities in social capital and health between people with and without disabilities', *Social Science & Medicine*, **126**, pp. 26-35. Available at: https://doi.org/10.1016/j.socscimed.2014.12.009.

Moss, S., Prosser, H., Costello, H., Simpson, N., Patel, P., Rowe, S., Turner, S., and Hatton, C. (1998) 'Reliability and validity of the PAS-ADD Checklist for detecting psychiatric disorders in adults with intellectual disability', *Journal of Intellectual Disability Research*, **42**(2), pp. 173-183. Available at: doi: 10.1046/j.1365-2788.1998.00116.x

National Health Service (2022) *Mindfulness*. Available at: https://www.nhs.uk/mental-health/self-help/tips-and-support/mindfulness/ (Accessed: 10 August 2023).

National Institute for Health and Care Excellence (2015) *Challenging behaviour and learning disabilities prevention and interventions for people with learning disabilities whose behaviour challenges*. Available at: https://www.nice.org.uk/guidance/ng11

Nind, M. and Hewett, D. (1994) *Access to Communication: Developing the Basics of Communication with People with Severe Learning Difficulties through Intensive Interaction*. London: David Fulton

Nirje, B. (1972) The right to self-determination. In W. Wolfensberger, *The principle of Normalization in human services*. Toronto: National Institute on Mental Retardation.

O'Brien, J. (2002) 'Person-Centered Planning as a Contributing Factor in Organizational and Social Change', *Research and Practice for Persons with Severe Disabilities*, **27**(4), pp. 261-264. Available at: https://doi.org/10.2511/rpsd.27.4.261

O'Brien, J. and O'Brien, C. L., (1991) *More that just new address: Images of organisation for supported living agencies*. Beverly Hills: Sage. Available at: https://inclusion.com/site/wp-content/uploads/2017/12/More-than-just-a-new-address.pdf

O'Brien, J., Pearpoint, J. and Kahn, L. (2010) *The PATH & MAPS Handbook: Person-Centered Ways to Build Community*. Toronto: Inclusion Press.

O'Leary, L., Cooper, S-A. and Hughes-McCormack, L. (2018) 'Early death and causes of death of people with intellectual disabilities: a systematic review', *Journal of Applied Research in Intellectual Disabilities*, **31**(3), pp. 325–42. Available at: DOI: 10.1111/jar.12417

O'Neill, R.E., Albin, R.W., Storey, K., Horner, R.H. and Sprague, J.R. (2015) *Functional assessment and program development*. Stamford: Cengage Learning.

Prosser, H., Moss, S., Costello, H., Simpson, N., Patel, P. and Rowe, S. (1997) 'Reliability and validity of the Mini PAS-ADD for assessing psychiatric disorders in adults with intellectual disability', *Journal of Intellectual Disability Research*, **42**(4), 264-272. Available at: doi: 10.1046/j.1365- 2788.1998.00146.x

Quilliam, C., Bigby, C. and Douglas, J. (2018) 'Being a valuable contributor on the frontline: The self-perception of staff in group homes for people with intellectual disability', *Journal of Applied Research in Intellectual Disabilities*, **31**(3), pp. 395-404. Available at: https://doi.org/10.1111/jar.12418

 Enabling Capable Environments © Pavilion Publishing and Media Ltd and its licensors 2024.

Ratti, V., Hassiotis, A., Crabtree, J., Deb, S., Gallagher, P. and Unwin, G. (2016) 'The effectiveness of person-centred planning for people with intellectual disabilities: A systematic review', *Research in Developmental Disabilities*, **57**, pp. 63–84. Available at: doi: 10.1016/j.ridd.2016.06.015.

Revell. A.J. and Ayotte, B.J. (2020) Novel Approaches to Teaching Aging and Disability: Active Learning Through Design and Exploration. *The International Journal of Aging and Human Development*, **91**(4), pp. 373-380. Available at: doi:10.1177/0091415020912944

Roy, A., Matthews, H., Clifford, P., Fowler, V. and Martin, D. (2002) 'Health of the Nation Outcome Scales for People with Learning Disabilities (HoNOS-LD)', *British Journal of Psychiatry*, **180**, pp. 61-66. Available at: DOI: 10.1192/bjp.180.1.61

Royal College of Psychiatrists, British Psychological Society and Royal College of Speech and Language Therapists. (2007) *Challenging behaviour: a unified approach [College Report No.144]*. London: Royal College of Psychiatrists.

Ryff, C.D. (1989) 'Happiness is everything, or is it? 'Explorations on the meaning of psychological well-being", *Journal of Personality and Social Psychology*, **57**(6), pp. 1069–1081. Available at: https://doi.org/10.1037/0022-3514.57.6.1069

Sailor, W., Dunlap, G,. Sugai, G. and Horner, R. (2010) *Handbook of Positive Behavior Support*. New York: Springer Science.

Sanderson, H. (2000) *Person Centred Planning: Key Features and Approaches*, Helen Sanderson Associates. Available at: https://proudtocaresurrey.org.uk/wp-content/uploads/2019/06/pcp-key-features-and-styles.pdf

Schalock, R.L. (2004) 'The concept of quality of life: What we know and do not know', *Journal of Intellectual Disability Research*, **48**(3), pp. 203–216. Available at: https://doi.org/10.1111/j.1365-2788.2003.00558.x

Schalock, R.L. and Alonso, M.A.V. (2015) 'The Impact of the Quality-of-Life Concept on the Field of Intellectual Disability', in M.L. Wehmeyer (Ed.), *The oxford handbook of positive psychology and disability*. New York: Oxford University Press, pp. 37-47.

Schalock, R.L., Brown, I., Brown, R., Cummins, R.A., Felce, D., Matikka, L., et al. (2002) 'Conceptualization, measurement, and application of quality of life for persons with intellectual disabilities: Report of an international panel of experts', *American Association on Mental Retardation*, **40**(6), pp. 457–470. Available at: DOI: 10.1352/0047-6765(2002)040<0457:CMAAOQ>2.0.CO;2

Schalock, R.L., Keith, K.D., Verdugo, M.Á. and Gómez, L.E. (2010) 'Quality of Life Model Development and Use in the Field of Intellectual Disability', in R. Kober (Ed.), *Enhancing the Quality of Life of People with Intellectual Disabilities: From Theory to Practice* [Online]. Springer Dordrecht, pp. 17.32. Available at: https://link.springer.com/book/10.1007/978-90-481-9650-0#about-this-book. (Accessed: 25 October 2023)

Schore, J.R. and Schore, A.N. (2008) 'Modern attachment theory: The central role of affect regulation in development and treatment', *Clinical Social Work Journal*, **36**(1), 9-20. Available at: https://doi.org/10.1007/s10615-007-0111-7

Scottish Executive. (2000) *The same as you? A review of services for people with learning disabilities*. Edinburgh: Scottish Executive.

Shapiro, S.L. (2020) *Rewire your mind: Discover the science & practice of mindfulness*. London: Aster.

Siegel, D.J. (2012) *The Developing Mind: How Relationships and the Brain Interact to Shape Who We Are*. Second edition. New York: The Guilford Press.

Singh, N.N., Lancioni, G.E., Medvedev, O.N. et al. (2020) 'Comparative Effectiveness of Caregiver Training in Mindfulness-Based Positive Behavior Support (MBPBS) and Positive Behavior Support (PBS) in a Randomized Controlled Trial', *Mindfulness*, **11**, pp. 99–111. Available at: https://doi.org/10.1007/s12671-018-0895-2

Singh, N.N., Lancioni, G.E., Winton, A.S.W., Singh, A.N., Adkins, A.D., and Singh, J. (2009) 'Mindful Staff Can Reduce the Use of Physical Restraints When Providing Care to Individuals with Intellectual Disabilities', *Journal of Applied Research in Intellectual Disabilities*, **22**(2), pp. 194–202. Available at: https://doi.org/10.1111/j.1468-3148.2008.00488.x

Skills for Care (2024) *Manager Induction Standards: Supporting and Developing Teams*. Available at: https://www.skillsforcare.org.uk/Support-for-leaders-and-managers/Developing-leaders-and-managers/Manager-induction-standards/2-Supporting-and-developing-teams.aspx (Accessed: 2 December 2023).

Skirrow, P. and Perry, E. (2009) *The Maslow Assessment of Needs Scales*. Mersey Care NHS Trust

Spicer, M. and Crates, N. (2016) 'Non-aversive reactive strategies for reducing the episodic severity of aggression', *International Journal of Positive Behavioural Support*, **6**(1), pp. 35–51. Available at: https://www.ingentaconnect.com/content/bild/ijpbs/2016/00000006/00000001/art00004

Stancliffe, R.J., Shogren, K.A. and Wehmeyer, M.L. (2020) 'Policies and Practices to Support Preference, Choice, and Self-Determination: An Ecological Understanding', in R.J. Stancliffe, M.L. Wehmeyer, K.A. Shogren. & B.H. Abery (Eds.), *Choice, Preference, and Disability: Promoting Self-Determination Across the Lifespan*. Switzerland: Springer Nature Switzerland AG, pp. 339-354.

Szabo, T., Williams, L., Rafacz, S.D. and Lydon, C. (2012) 'Evaluation of the Service Review Model with Performance Scorecards', *Journal of Organizational Behavior Management*, **34**(4), pp. 274-296. Available at: doi: 10.1080/01608061.2012.729408.

The British Institute of Human Rights (2016) *Learning Disability and Human Rights: A practitioner's guide*. Available at: https://knowyourhumanrights.co.uk/resources/BIHR_Mental_Health_Practitioner_Resource_LearningDisability.pdf

The Challenging Behaviour Foundation (2020) *Broken: The psychological trauma suffered by family carers of children and adults with a learning disability and / or autism and the support required. The Challenging Behaviour Foundation Report*. Available at: https://www.challengingbehaviour.org.uk/wp-content/uploads/2021/03/brokencbffinalreportstrand1jan21.pdf (Accessed 21 May 23).

The Chartered Institute for Personnel and Development (2023) *Stress in the Workplace*. Available at: https://www.cipd.org/uk/knowledge/factsheets/stress-factsheet/#:~:text=Stress%20can%20place%20immense%20demands,key%20to%20managing%20people%20effectively (Accessed: 22 November 2023).

Topping, M., Douglas, J. and Winkler, D. (2022) '" They treat you like a person , they ask you what you want ": a grounded theory study of quality paid disability support for adults with acquired neurological disability', *Disability and Rehabilitation*, **45**(13) pp. 2138–2148. Available at: doi: 10.1080/09638288.2022.2086636.

Totsika, V., Toogood, S. and Hastings, R.P. (2008) 'Active support: Development, evidence base, and future directions', *Review of Research in Mental Retardation*, **35**, pp. 205-249. Available at: DOI: 10.1016/S0074-7750(07)35006-4

 Enabling Capable Environments © Pavilion Publishing and Media Ltd and its licensors 2024.

Turner, S. and Harder, N. (2018) Psychological Safe Environment: A Concept Analysis. *Clinical Simulation in Nursing*, (18), pp. 47-55. Available at: https://doi.org/10.1016/j.ecns.2018.02.004.

United Nations (2006) *Convention on the Rights of Persons with Disabilities*. Available at: http://www.un.org/disabilities/convention/conventionfull.shtml

United Response and Tizard Centre (2016) *'What does good look like? A guide for observing in services for people with learning disabilities and / or autism'*. Available at: https://www.unitedresponse.org.uk/resource/what-does-good-look-like/ (Accessed on 12th January 2024)

Ward, T. and Brown, M. (2004) 'The Good Lives Model and conceptual issues in offender rehabilitation', *Psychology, Crime & Law*, **10** (3), pp. 243-257. https://doi.org/10.1080/10683160410001662744

Wehmeyer, M. L. (2020) 'The Importance of Self-Determination to the Quality of Life of People with Intellectual Disability: A Perspective', *International Journal of Environmental Research and Public Health*, **17**(19), pp. 7121. Available at: https://doi.org/10.3390/ijerph17197121

West, M. (2021) in Bailey, S., and West, M. (2022) *What is Compassionate Leadership?* Available at: https://www.kingsfund.org.uk/publications/what-is-compassionate-leadership. (Accessed: 4 January 2024).

West, M., Armit, K., Loewenthal, L., Eckert, R., West, T. and Lee, A. (2015) *Leadership and leadership development in health care: the evidence base*. London. The King's Fund.

West, M. and Dawson, J. (2012) in Bailey, S., and West, M. (2022) *What is Compassionate Leadership?* Available at: https://www.kingsfund.org.uk/publications/what-is-compassionate-leadership (Accessed: 4 January 2024)

World Health Organization (2016) *Framework on Integrated, People-centred Health Services. Report by the Secretariat*. Available at: https://apps.who.int/gb/ebwha/pdf_files/WHA69/A69_39-en.pdf

World Health Organization (2020) *Disability*. Available at: https://www.who.int/news-room/fact-sheets/detail/disability-and-health.